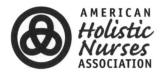

AMERICAN
Holistic
Nurses
ASSOCIATION

W9-BEA-265

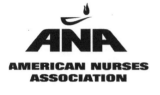

AMERICAN NURSES
ASSOCIATION

Scope AND
Standards
OF PRACTICE

Holistic

Nursing

2ND EDITION

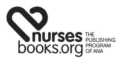

nurses THE
PUBLISHING
books.org PROGRAM
OF ANA

American Nurses Association
Silver Spring, Maryland
2013

American Nurses Association
8515 Georgia Avenue, Suite 400
Silver Spring, MD 20910-3492
1-800-274-4ANA
http://www.NursingWorld.org

Published by Nursesbooks.org
The Publishing Program of ANA
http://www.Nursesbooks.org/

The American Holistic Nurses Association (AHNA) and the American Nurses Association (ANA) are national professional associations. This joint ANA–AHNA publication—*Holistic Nursing: Scope and Standards of Practice, 2nd Edition*—reflects the thinking of the practice specialty of holistic nursing on various issues and should be reviewed in conjunction with state board of nursing policies and practices. State law, rules, and regulations govern the practice of nursing, while *Holistic Nursing: Scope and Standards of Practice, 2nd Edition* guides holistic nurses in the application of their professional skills and responsibilities.

About the American Nurses Association
The American Nurses Association (ANA) is the only full-service professional organization representing the interests of the nation's 3.1 million registered nurses through its constituent/state nurses associations and its organizational affiliates. The ANA advances the nursing profession by fostering high standards of nursing practice, promoting the rights of nurses in the workplace, projecting a positive and realistic view of nursing, and by lobbying the Congress and regulatory agencies on health care issues affecting nurses and the public.

About the American Holistic Nurses Association
The American Holistic Nurses Association (AHNA) is a nonprofit membership organization that is open to nurses and other individuals interested in holistically oriented health care practices throughout the United States and the world. Founded in 1981, AHNA is the definitive voice for holistic nursing and supports the education of nurses, allied health practitioners, and the general public on health-related issues and the concepts of holism: a state of harmony among body, mind, emotions, and spirit within an ever-changing environment.

ISBN-13: 978-1-55810-478-5   SAN: 851-3481   11/2014R

First printing: February 2013. Second Printing: November 2014.

Contents

Contributors

Primary Contributor:
Carla Mariano, EdD, RN, AHN-BC, FAAIM

The work of many provided the foundation for *Holistic Nursing: Scope and Standards of Practice* (2007) and its evolution into this, the second edition (2013). These are cited in Appendix A and throughout the document. Most notable are: Barbara Montgomery Dossey, PhD, RN, AHN-BC, FAAN; Noreen Cavan Frisch, PhD, RN, AHN-BC, FAAN; Lynn Keegan, PhD, RN, AHN-BC, FAAN; Carla Mariano, EdD, RN, AHN-BC, FAAIM; Jean Watson, PhD, RN, AHN-BC, FAAN.

The Task Forces and Review Committees, for the following documents:

- *Holistic Nursing: Scope and Standards of Practice* (2007)

- *Standards of Holistic Nursing Practice* (2005)

- *Standards of Advanced Holistic Practice for Graduate-Prepared Nurses* (2005)

- AHNA Position Statements and White Papers

Other key contributors: the Leadership Councils and Staff of the American Holistic Nurses Association (AHNA), Charlotte McGuire, and the founding members of the AHNA. And, the numerous holistic nurses throughout the years who have contributed to the body of holistic nursing knowledge and advancement of the specialty of holistic nursing in practice, research, education, certification, administration, advocacy, and health care.

Finally, sincere appreciation to Carol Bickford, PhD, RN-BC, Senior Policy Fellow, American Nurses Association, for your wise and helpful suggestions, your support during the process, and your belief in holistic nursing.

CM

American Nurses Association Staff

Carol Bickford, PhD, RN-BC, CPHIMS—Content editor

Maureen E. Cones, Esq.—Legal counsel

Yvonne Daley Humes, MSA—Project coordinator

Eric Wurzbacher, BA—Project editor

About the American Holistic Nurses Association

The American Holistic Nurses Association (AHNA) is a nonprofit membership organization that is open to nurses and other individuals interested in holistically oriented health care practices throughout the United States and the world. Founded in 1981, is the definitive voice for holistic nursing and supports the education of nurses, allied health practitioners, and the general public on health-related issues and the concepts of holism: a state of harmony among body, mind, emotions, and spirit within an ever-changing environment.

About the American Nurses Association

The American Nurses Association (ANA) is the only full-service professional organization representing the interests of the nation's 3.1 million registered nurses through its constituent/state nurses associations and its organizational affiliates. The ANA advances the nursing profession by fostering high standards of nursing practice, promoting the rights of nurses in the workplace, projecting a positive and realistic view of nursing, and by lobbying the Congress and regulatory agencies on healthcare issues affecting nurses and the public.

About Nursesbooks.org, The Publishing Program of ANA

Nursesbooks.org publishes books on ANA core issues and programs, including ethics, leadership, quality, specialty practice, advanced practice, and the profession's enduring legacy. Best known for the foundational documents of the profession on nursing ethics, scope and standards of practice, and social policy, Nursesbooks.org is the publisher for the professional, career-oriented nurse, reaching and serving nurse educators, administrators, managers, and researchers as well as staff nurses in the course of their professional development.

Introduction

Extraordinary changes have occurred in health care and nursing during the past decade. The purpose of this document is to articulate the scope and standards of the specialty practice of holistic nursing and to inform holistic nurses, the nursing profession, other healthcare providers and disciplines, employers, third-party payers, legislators, and the public about the unique scope of knowledge and the standards of practice and professional performance of a holistic nurse.

Holistic Nursing: Scope and Standards of Practice, 2nd Edition, is the foundational document and resource for holistic nursing education at all levels (undergraduate, graduate, continuing education), and for holistic nursing practice, research, advocacy, and certification.

Function of the Scope of Practice Statement of Holistic Nursing

The scope of practice statement describes the *who, what, where, when, why,* and *how* of the practice of holistic nursing. The answers to these questions provide a picture of the dynamic and complex practice of holistic nursing, its evolving boundaries, and its membership.

Nursing: Scope and Standards of Practice, 2nd Edition (ANA, 2010b) applies to all professional registered nurses engaged in practice, regardless of specialty, practice setting, or educational preparation. With the *Guide to the Code of Ethics for Nurses: Interpretation and Application* (ANA, 2010a) and *Nursing's Social Policy Statement: The Essence of the Profession* (ANA, 2010c), it forms the foundation of practice for all registered nurses. The scope of holistic nursing practice is specific to this specialty, but it builds on the scope of practice expected of all registered nurses.

Function of the Standards of Holistic Nursing

"The Standards of Professional Nursing Practice are authoritative statements of the duties that all registered nurses, regardless of role, population, or specialty, are expected to perform competently. The standards published herein may serve as evidence of the standard of care, with the understanding that application of the standards depends on context. The standards are subject to change with the dynamics of the nursing profession, as new patterns of professional practice are developed and accepted by the nursing profession and the public. In addition, specific conditions and clinical circumstances may also affect the application of the standards at a given time" (ANA, 2010b, p. 2). "[S]tandards reflect the values and priorities of the profession. Standards provide direction for professional nursing practice and a framework for evaluation of this practice. Written in measurable terms, these standards define the nursing profession's accountability to the public and the outcomes for which registered nurses are responsible" (ANA, 2004, p. 1). The standards of holistic nursing practice are specific to this specialty, but build on the standards of practice expected of all registered nurses.

Function of Competencies Accompanying Standards of Holistic Nursing

A *competency* is "[a]n expected and measureable level of nursing performance that integrates knowledge, skills, abilities, and judgment, based on established scientific knowledge and expectations for nursing practice" (ANA, 2010b, p. 64). The competencies that accompany each standard in this book are evidence of compliance with the corresponding standard. The list of competencies is not exhaustive and may depend on circumstances or context.

Development of the Holistic Nursing Standards of Practice: Basic and Advanced

The American Holistic Nurses Association (AHNA) first developed *Standards of Holistic Nursing Practice* in 1990. [See Appendix A, *Holistic Nursing: Scope and Standards of Practice* (2007), for the development of the original *Standards of Holistic Nursing Practice* and the *Standards of Advanced Holistic Nursing for Graduate Prepared Nurses.*] In 2006, holistic nursing was officially recognized by the American Nurses Association (ANA) as a distinct specialty within nursing. The first edition of *Holistic Nursing:*

Scope and Standards of Practice was jointly published by the AHNA and ANA in 2007.

Summary

Holistic Nursing: Scope and Standards of Practice, 2nd Edition (2013) reflects a consensus of the most current thinking in the specialty and provides a blueprint for holistic nursing philosophy, principles, and practices. It incorporates the fundamental philosophical beliefs and practices as well as new developments and advancements in the field of holistic nursing. It is the foundational, key resource for education, practice, research, advocacy, and certification in holistic nursing. This document guides clinicians, educators, researchers, nurse managers, and administrators in professional activities, knowledge, and performance that are relevant to basic and advanced practice, education, research, and advocacy in holistic nursing.

Holistic Nursing Scope of Practice

Definition and Overview of Holistic Nursing

Holistic nursing is defined as "all nursing practice that has healing the whole person as its goal" (AHNA, 1998).

Holistic nursing focuses on protecting, promoting, and optimizing health and wellness; assisting healing; preventing illness and injury; alleviating suffering; supporting people to find peace, comfort, harmony, and balance through the diagnosis and treatment of human response; and advocacy in the care of individuals, families, communities, populations, and the planet.

Holistic nursing embraces all nursing that has the enhancement of healing the whole person from birth to death—and all age groups from infant to elder—as its goal. This means viewing the whole person and his/her needs in their entirety, with integration as the goal. The holistic nurse recognizes and integrates body-mind-emotion-spirit-energetic-environment principles and modalities in daily life and clinical practice; creates a caring healing space within herself/himself that allows the nurse to be an instrument of healing; shares authenticity of unconditional presence that helps to remove the barriers to the healing process; facilitates another person's growth (body-mind-emotion-spirit-energetic-environment connections); and assists with maintaining wellness, recovery from illness, or transition to peaceful death.

Holistic nursing honors the interconnectedness of self, others, nature, and spirituality. Holistic nursing recognizes that there are two views regarding holism: that holism involves identifying the interrelationships of a person's bio-psycho-social-spiritual dimensions, recognizing that the whole is greater than the sum of its parts; and that holism involves understanding the individual as a unitary whole in mutual process with the environment. Holistic nursing responds to both views, believing that the goals of nursing can be achieved within either framework.

Holistic nursing care is person and relationship centered and healing oriented, rather than disease and cure oriented. Holistic nursing emphasizes

1

practices of self-care, intentionality, presence, mindfulness, and therapeutic use of self as pivotal for facilitation of healing and patterning of wellness in others. Holistic nursing is prospective, focusing on:

- Comprehensive health promotion and disease and illness risk reduction.

- Proactive interventions that address antecedents and mediators of disease.

- Opportunities in each individual's experiences of illness and disease for the individual's transformation, growth, and finding of meaning.

The holistic nurse is an instrument of healing and a facilitator in the healing process. Holistic nurses honor the individual's subjective experience about health, health beliefs, and values. To allow nurses to become therapeutic partners with individuals, families, communities, and populations, holistic nursing practice draws on nursing knowledge, theories, research, expertise, intuition, and creativity, incorporating the roles of clinician, educator, consultant, coach, partner, role model, and advocate. Holistic nursing practice encourages peer review of professional practice in various clinical settings and provides care based on current professional standards, laws, and regulations governing nursing practice.

Philosophically, holistic nursing is a worldview—a way of being in the world, not just the use of modalities. Holistic nurses do incorporate complementary/alternative/integrative modalities (CAM) into clinical practice to treat people's physiological, psychological, and spiritual needs. Doing so does not negate the validity of conventional medical therapies, but rather serves to complement, broaden, and enrich the scope of nursing practice and to help individuals access their greatest healing potential. Assimilation of a holistic philosophy and various healing practices is advocated rather than separation/fragmentation.

Practicing holistic nursing requires nurses to integrate self-reflection, self-care, self-responsibility, and spirituality in their own lives and to serve as role-models to others. This leads the nurse to greater awareness of the interconnectedness with oneself, others, nature, and God/LifeForce/Absolute/Transcendent. This awareness further enhances nurses' understanding of all individuals and their relationships to the human and global community, and it permits nurses to use this awareness to facilitate the healing process.

The phenomena of concern to holistic nursing include, but are not limited to:

- The caring–healing relationship

- The subjective experience of and meanings ascribed to health, illness, wellness, healing, birth, growth and development, and dying

- The cultural values and beliefs and folk practices of health, illness, and healing

- Physical, mental, emotional, and spiritual comfort, discomfort, and pain

- Spirituality in nursing care

- Energy and consciousness

- Reflective practice

- The use and evaluation of complementary/alternative/integrative modalities in nursing practice

- Comprehensive health promotion, disease prevention, and well-being

- Self-care processes

- Empowerment, decision-making, and the ability to make informed choices

- Social and economic policies and their effects on the health of individuals, families, and communities

- Diverse and alternative healthcare systems and their relationships to access and quality of health care

- Healing environments

- The environment, ecosystem, and the prevention of disease

This document, used in conjunction with *Nursing's Social Policy Statement: The Essence of the Profession* (ANA, 2010c), *Nursing: Scope and Standards of Practice, 2nd Edition* (ANA, 2010b), *Guide to the Code of Ethics for Nurses: Interpretation and Application* (ANA, 2010a), and the laws, statutes, and regulations related to nursing practice for the nurse's state, commonwealth, or territory, delineates the professional responsibilities of a holistic nurse.

Evolution of Holistic Nursing

"Holism" in health care is a philosophy that emanated directly from Florence Nightingale, who believed in care that focused on unity, wellness, and the interrelationship of human beings, events, and environment. She "clearly articulated the science and art of an integrated worldview for nursing, health care, and humankind" (Dossey, 2010). Even Hippocrates, the father of Western medicine, espoused a holistic orientation when he taught doctors to observe their patients' life circumstances and emotional states. Socrates stated, "Curing the soul; that is the first thing." In holism, symptoms are believed to be an expression of the body's wisdom as it reacts to cure its own imbalance or dis-ease.

The root of the word *heal* comes from the Greek word *halos* and the Anglo-Saxon word *healan*, which means "to be or to become whole." The word *holy* also comes from the same source. Healing means "making whole"—or restoring balance and harmony. It is movement toward a sense of wholeness and completion. Healing therefore is the integration of the totality of the person in body, mind, emotion, spirit, energy, and environment.

One of the driving forces behind the holistic nursing movement in the United States was the formation of the American Holistic Nurses Association (AHNA) in 1980 by Charlotte McGuire and 75 founding members. AHNA, the definitive voice for holistic nursing, is a nonprofit membership association for nurses and other holistic healthcare professionals, promoting the education of nurses, other healthcare professionals, and the public in all aspects of holistic caring, healing, and integrative health care.

Membership in AHNA has almost doubled in the past 5 years; AHNA now serves more than 5,700 members, 146 local chapters across the United States, and an international membership from 14 countries. AHNA has as its focus uniting nurses in healing, with an emphasis on holistic principles of health, preventive education, and the integration of allopathic and complementary caring–healing modalities to facilitate care of the whole person and significant others. AHNA's vision is "a world in which nursing nurtures wholeness and inspires peace and healing" and its mission is "to advance holistic nursing through community building, advocacy, research, and education." From its inception, the American Holistic Nurses Association has been the leader in developing and advancing holistic principles, practices, and guidelines. AHNA predicted that holistic principles, caring–healing, and the integration of complementary/alternative/integrative therapies would merge into mainstream health care.

AHNA is committed to promoting wholeness and wellness in individuals, families, communities, nurses themselves, the nursing profession, and the environment. Through its various activities, AHNA provides vision, direction, and leadership in the advancement of holistic nursing; integrates the art and science of nursing into the profession; serves as a supportive community and resource to members; empowers holistic nursing through education, research, and standards; promotes research and scholarship in the field of holistic nursing; encourages nurses to be models of wellness; honors individual excellence in the advancement of holistic nursing; and influences policy to change the healthcare system to a more humanistic orientation. (See Appendix B for the AHNA goals and activities.)

The relevance and validity of holistic nursing as a science and practice has been increasingly demonstrated in recent years. "While becoming more popular and more highly regarded, holism and holistic nursing have contributed to enhancing the human condition in many ways. Holism as a philosophy, concept, theory, and practice has been used to expand our understanding of human wellness and illness. Holistic nursing has become more systematized, refined, and diversified as strategies and practices have been shown to have an impact on health and well-being. Holistic nursing has progressed through the development of standards, endorsement of programs, and certification of beginning and advanced practitioners. Holistic nursing's contributions to human welfare have been increasingly recognized . . . as evidenced by their current standing in healthcare and appreciation by society. . . . [H]olism as a perspective and holistic nursing as a response may offer the world something that counteracts the fragmentation and isolation that exists so predominantly in our society. . . . [H]olistic nursing provides a context in which nurses can consider, understand, and appreciate all the aspects of human experience that contribute to patterns of life, health, and illness" (Cowling, 2011, p. 5).

There has been a substantial increase in the numbers of holistic nurses who hold leadership roles as clinicians, educators, administrators, consultants, authors, and researchers in practice environments, university-based schools of nursing, and nursing and other professional organizations.

Philosophical Principles of Holistic Nursing

Holistic nurses express, contribute to, and promote an understanding of:

- A philosophy of nursing that values healing as the desired outcome

- The human health experience as a complex, dynamic relationship of health, illness, disease, and wellness

- The scientific foundations of nursing practice; and nursing as an art

The following philosophical principles—Person, Healing/Health, Practice, Nursing Roles, and Self-Reflection and Self-Care—serve as the framework for holistic nursing.

Person

- There is unity, totality, and connectedness of everyone and everything (body, mind, emotion, spirit, sexuality, age, environment, social/cultural, belief systems, relationships, context, energy).

- Human beings are unique, diverse, and inherently good.

- People are able to find meaning and purpose in their own life, experiences, and illness.

- All people have an innate power and capacity for self-healing. Health/illness is subjectively described and determined by the view of the individual. Therefore, the person is honored in all phases of his/her healing process regardless of expectations or outcomes.

- People/persons/individuals are the recipients of holistic nursing services. They may be healthcare consumers, clients, patients, families, significant others, populations, or communities. They may be ill and within the healthcare delivery system, or well and moving toward personal betterment and enhanced well-being.

Healing/Health

- Health and illness are natural and a part of life, learning, and movement toward change and development.

- Health is seen as balance, integration, harmony, right relationship, and the betterment of well-being, not just the absence of disease. Healing can take place without cure. The focus is on health promotion/disease prevention/health restoration/lifestyle patterns and habits, as well as symptom relief.

- Illness is considered a teacher, an opportunity for self-awareness and growth, and part of the life process. Symptoms are respected as messages.

- Healing is multidimensional, can occur at any level of the human system, and is creative, unfolding, and unpredictable.

- People as active partners in the healing process are empowered when they take some control of their own lives, health, and well-being, including personal choices and relationships.

■ Treatment is a process that considers the root of the problem/issue/illness, not merely treating the obvious signs and symptoms.

Practice

■ Practice is a science (critical thinking, reflection, evidence/research/theory as foundational to practice) and an art (intuition, creativity, appreciation, presence, self/personal knowing as integral to practice).

■ The values and ethic of holism, caring, moral insight, dignity, integrity, competence, responsibility, accountability, and legality underlie holistic nursing practice.

■ Intention for the well-being and highest good of the care recipient is the cornerstone of all holistic practice.

■ Any and all interventions affect the whole.

■ There are various philosophies and paradigms of health, illness, healing, and wellness, and approaches/models for the delivery of health care (both in the United States and in other cultures) that should be understood and utilized.

■ Older adults represent the predominant population served by nurses.

■ Public policy and the healthcare delivery system influence the health and well-being of society and professional nursing.

Nursing Roles

Nursing roles include:

■ Using warmth, compassion, caring, authenticity, respect, trust, and relationship as instruments of healing in and of themselves, and as part of the healing environment.

■ Using conventional nursing interventions as well as holistic/complementary/alternative/integrative modalities that enhance body-mind-emotion-spirit-environment connectedness to foster healing, health, wholeness, and well-being of people.

■ Collaborating and partnering with all constituencies in the health process, including the person receiving care, family, significant others, community, peers, and other disciplines. This involves using principles and skills of cooperation, alliance, and consensus, and respecting and honoring the contributions of all.

■ Participating in the change process to develop more caring cultures in which to practice, learn, and live.

■ Assisting nurses to nurture and heal themselves.

■ Participating in activities that contribute to the improvement of local and global communities, as well as the betterment of public health, the environment, and the planet.

■ Acting as an advocate for the rights of and equitable distribution of and access to health care for all persons, especially vulnerable populations.

■ Participating in the positive transformation of systems.

■ Honoring the ecosystem and our relationship with and need to preserve it, as we are all connected.

Self-Reflection and Self-Care

■ Self-reflection—defined as turning inward to examine one's thoughts, values, beliefs, experiences, behaviors, and inner wisdom—enhances self-understanding and facilitates reflective practice.

■ The nurse's self-reflection, self-assessment, self-care, healing, and personal development are necessary for service to others, growth/change in the nurse's own well-being, and understanding of the nurse's own personal journey.

■ The nurse values herself/himself and her/his calling to holistic nursing as a life purpose.

Integrating the Art and Science of Nursing: Core Values

The art and science of holistic nursing emanates from the following five core values, which are described in this section:

■ Core Value 1. Holistic Philosophy, Theories, and Ethics

■ Core Value 2. Holistic Caring Process

- Core Value 3. Holistic Communication, Therapeutic Healing Environment, and Cultural Diversity

- Core Value 4. Holistic Education and Research

- Core Value 5. Holistic Nurse Self-Reflection and Self-Care

Core Value 1. Holistic Philosophy, Theories, and Ethics

Philosophical, theoretical, and ethical foundations define the *who* and *why* of holistic nursing—who holistic nurses are and their raison d'être.

Holistic nurses recognize the human health experience as a complicated, dynamic relationship of health, illness, and wellness, and they value healing as the desired outcome of the practice of nursing. Their practice is based on both scientific foundations (theory, research, evidence-based/informed practice, critical thinking, reflection) and art (relationship, communication, creativity, presence, caring).

Holistic nursing is grounded in nursing knowledge and skill and guided by nursing theory. Florence Nightingale's writings are often referenced as a significant precursor for the development of holistic nursing practice. Although each holistic nurse chooses which nursing theory to apply in any individual case, the nursing theories of Jean Watson (Theory of Human Caring and Caring Science), Martha Rogers (Science of Unitary Human Beings), Margaret Newman (Health as Expanding Consciousness), Madeleine Leininger (Theory of Cultural Care Diversity and Universality), Hildegard Peplau (Theory of Interpersonal Relations), Rosemarie Rizzo Parse (Human Becoming School of Thought), Josephine Paterson and Loretta Zderad (Humanistic Nursing Theory), and Helen Erickson, Evelyn Tomlin, and Mary Ann Swain (Modeling and Role-Modeling) are most frequently used to support holistic nursing practice.

There has been significant development in the evolution of holism, healing, and caring conceptualization and theory, much done by holistic nurses. Prominent among those are Barbara Dossey (Theory of Integral Nursing), Marlaine Smith (Theory of Unitary Caring), Marilyn Anne Ray (Theory of Bureaucratic Caring), Rozzano Locsin (Technological Competency as Caring and the Practice of Knowing Persons in Nursing), Mary Jane Smith and Patricia Liehr (Story Theory), and Joanne Duffy (Quality Caring Model). Additionally, the International Association for Human Caring (IAHC), of which many holistic nurses are members and leaders, is an international organization that provides the forum for discovery and dissemination of caring science; identifies major philosophical, epistemological, and professional dimensions of care and caring to advance the body of knowledge; assists nursing and other disciplines to use care and caring knowledge in human relationships and to facilitate the application of this knowledge to transform organizational systems in which nurses function to become care-focused; stimulates nurse scholars and other professionals worldwide to systematically investigate care and caring and to share findings with colleagues at an annual research conference and through refereed publications and public forums.

In addition to nursing theory, holistic nurses utilize other theories and perspectives of wholeness and healing to guide their practice. These scientific theories and philosophies present a worldview of connectedness, and include theories of consciousness; systems theory; energy field theory; quantum physics; complexity science; chaos theory; coherence; Carl Pribram's Holographic Universe; David Bohm's Implicate/Explicate Order; psychoneuroimmunology; Rupert Sheldrake's Morphic Resonance; Ken Wilbur's Integral Theory; various philosophical perspectives such as Pierre Tielhard de Chardin's philosophy; spirituality; and alternative medical systems such as traditional oriental medicine, traditional Chinese medicine, Ayurveda, Native American and indigenous healing, and Eastern contemplative orientations such as Zen Buddhism and Taoism.

Holistic nurses further recognize and honor the ethic that the person is the authority on his/her own health experience. The holistic nurse is an "option giver" who helps the person develop an understanding of alternatives and implications of various health and treatment options.

The holistic nurse first ascertains what the individual thinks or believes is happening to and with him or her, and then assists the person to identify what will help his/her situation. The assessment begins from where the individual is. The holistic nurse then discusses options, including the person's choices, across a continuum, including possible effects and implications of each choice. For instance, if a person diagnosed with cancer is experiencing nausea due to chemotherapy, the individual and nurse may discuss the choices and effects of pharmacologic agents, imagery, homeopathic remedies, and so forth, or a combination of these. The holistic nurse acts as partner and co-prescriptor rather than as a sole prescriber. The relationship is a co-piloting of the individual's health experience in which the nurse respects the person's decision about his/her own health. It is a process of engagement rather than compliance.

Client narratives, whether they arise from individuals, families, or communities, provide the context of the experiences and are used as an important focus in understanding the person's situation. Holistic nurses believe that people, through their inherent capacities, heal themselves. Therefore, the holistic nurse is not the "healer," but instead acts as a guide and facilitator of the individual's own healing.

In the belief that all things are connected, the holistic perspective espouses that an individual's actions have a ripple effect throughout humanity. Holism places the greatest worth on individuals' developing higher levels of human awareness and finding unity and wholeness within one's self, within humanity, and within nature. This, in turn, elevates the whole of humanity. Holistic nurses believe in the sacredness of one's self and of all nature. One's inner self and the collective greater self have stewardship not only over one's body, mind, and spirit, but also over our planet. Holistic nurses focus on the meaning and quality of life as derived from their own character and from their relationship to the universe, rather than as being imposed from outside the self.

Holistic nurses embrace a professional ethic of caring and healing that seeks to preserve the wholeness and dignity of self and others. They support human dignity by advocating and adhering to *The Patient's Bill of Rights in Medicare and Medicaid* (U.S. Department of Health and Human Services, 1999), ANA's *Guide to the Code of Ethics for Nurses: Interpretation and Application* (ANA, 2010a), and AHNA's *Position Statement on Holistic Nursing Ethics* (2012), the latter of which is included in Appendix D in this book.

Core Value 2. Holistic Caring Process

The holistic caring process identifies *what* holistic nurses do—that is, the practice of holistic nursing.

Holistic nurses provide care that recognizes the totality of the human being (the interconnectedness of body, mind, emotion, spirit, social/cultural, relationships, context, environment, and energy). This is an *integrated* as well as a comprehensive approach. While physical symptoms are being treated, a holistic nurse also focuses on how the individual is cognitively perceiving and emotionally dealing with the illness; its effect on the person's family, social relationships, and economic resources; the person's values and cultural/spiritual beliefs and preferences regarding treatment; and the meaning of this experience to the person's life. In addition, a holistic nurse may also incorporate a number of complementary/alternative/integrative modalities (e.g., cognitive restructuring, stress management, visualization and imagery, hypnotherapy, aromatherapy, Therapeutic Touch, Healing Touch) along with conventional nursing interventions. Holistic nurses focus on integrative care interventions that promote healing, peace, comfort, and a subjective sense of well-being for the person.

The holistic caring process is an iterative process that involves six steps, which often occur simultaneously: assessment, diagnosis (identification of pattern/problem/need/issue), outcomes identification, therapeutic plan of care, implementation, and evaluation. Holistic nurses apply the holistic caring process with individuals or families across the lifespan, population groups, and communities, and in all settings.

Holistic nurses take on a variety of roles in their practice, including those of expert clinician and facilitator of healing; consultant and collaborator; educator, coach, and guide; administrator, leader, and change agent; researcher; and advocate. They strongly emphasize partnership with individuals throughout the entire decision-making process.

Holistic assessments include not only the physical, functional, psychosocial, mental, emotional, cultural, and sexual aspects, but also spiritual, transpersonal, and energy-field assessments of the whole person. In today's world of reliance on electronic devices, energy forces and impacts become very important in understanding the health of both the human and the environment. Energy assessments are based on the concept that all beings are composed of energy. Congestion or stagnation of energy in any realm creates dis-harmony and dis-ease. Holistic nurses continuously use their necessary understanding of energy anatomy, electromagnetic fields, electromagnetic vibration, electromagnetic induction, and entrainment, not only in assessments but also in the healing process.

Spiritual assessments not only glean religious beliefs and practices, but also query a person's meaning and purpose in life and how that may have changed due to the present health experience. Spiritual assessments include questions about an individual's sense of serenity and peace, what provides joy and fulfillment, and the source of strength and hope.

Holistic assessment data are interpreted into patterns/challenges/needs from which meaning and understanding of the health/disease experience can be mutually identified with the person. An important responsibility is that of helping the person to identify risk factors such as lifestyle, habits, beliefs and values, personal and family health history, and age-related conditions that influence health and then to utilize opportunities to increase well-being. The focus is on the individual's goals, not the nurse's goals.

Therapeutic plans of care respect the person's experience and the uniqueness of each healing journey. The same illness may have very different manifestations in different individuals. A major aspect of holistic nursing practice, in addition to competence, is *intention*—that is, intending for the wholeness, well-being, and highest good of the person with every encounter and intervention. This honors and reinforces the innate capacity of people to heal themselves. Therefore, holistic nurses respect that outcomes may not be those expected and may evolve differently based on the person's own individual healing process and health choices.

Holistic nurses endeavor to detach themselves from the outcomes—or "let go of the ego." The nurse does not produce the outcomes; the individual's own healing process produces the outcomes, and the nurse facilitates this process. A significant focus is on guiding individuals and significant others to utilize their own inner strength and resources through the course of healing.

Appropriate and evidence-based information (including current knowledge, practice, and research) regarding the health condition and various treatments and therapies and their side effects is consistently provided. Holistic care always occurs within the scope and standards of practice of registered nursing and in accordance with state and federal laws and regulations.

In addition to conventional interventions, holistic nurses have knowledge of and integrate a number of CAM approaches, which have been categorized by the National Center for Complementary and Alternative Medicine (2011a). (See also Appendix C.) These categories include:

- Natural products, such as herbal therapies, diet therapies, nutritional supplements, and vitamins

- Mind–body interventions, such as meditation, relaxation, imagery, hypnosis, yoga, tai chi, prayer, art and music therapies, cognitive-behavioral therapy, biofeedback, therapeutic counseling, and stress management

- Manipulative and body-based methods, such as chiropractic, massage therapy, osteopathy, and reflexology

- Movement therapies, such as Feldenkrais method, Alexander Technique, Pilates, Rolfing, and dance therapy

- Practices of traditional indigenous healers, such as Native American, African, Middle Eastern, Tibetan, and Latin American

- Whole medical systems, such as Ayurveda, traditional Chinese medicine, traditional oriental medicine, homeopathy, and naturopathy

- Energy therapies, such as Therapeutic Touch, Reiki, qi gong, acupressure, Healing Touch, light therapy, and magnet therapy

Therapies frequently incorporated in holistic nursing practice include the following interventions listed in the 2008 Nursing Interventions Classification (NIC, n.d.): meditation; relaxation therapy; music, art, aroma, and activity therapies; energy-based touch therapies such as Therapeutic Touch and Healing Touch; acupressure; massage; guided imagery; hypnosis, animal-assisted therapy; biofeedback; humor; anxiety reduction and stress management; calming technique; emotional support, coping enhancement, and resiliency promotion; promotion of beneficial exercise, sleep, diet, and nutrition; energy management; substance use prevention; smoking cessation promotion; patient contracting; presence; journaling and bibliotherapy; self-awareness and body image enhancement; counseling; relationship building; cognitive therapy; self-help; forgiveness facilitation; hope inspiration; spiritual growth, support, and prayer; behavioral management and modification; resiliency promotion, conflict mediation and crisis intervention; risk identification; coaching; mutual goal setting and decision-making support; values clarification; reminiscence; pain management; dying care and grief work; family, support system, and caregiver support; support groups; anticipatory guidance, health education, learning facilitation and teaching; consultation, referral, health systems guidance, and cultural brokerage; community health development; and environmental management. Other interventions frequently employed in holistic nursing practice, in addition to conventional nursing interventions, include breath work, Reiki, reflexology, herbology and homeopathy, and Emotional Freedom Technique or Tapping.

Because many of today's healthcare problems (80% of all U.S. healthcare issues) are related to stress, holistic nurses empower individuals by teaching them techniques to reduce their stress. Many interventions used in holistic nursing elicit the relaxation response (e.g., breath work, meditation, relaxation, imagery, aromatherapy and use of essential oils, diet). People can learn these therapies and use them without the intervention of a healthcare provider, thereby empowering a person in his/her own healing and allowing the person to take an active role in the management of his/her own health care. Holistic nurses also can teach families and caregivers to use these techniques for loved ones who may be ill (e.g., simple foot or hand massage for older clients with dementia), fostering a sense of usefulness and supportive caring for their loved one. In addition, individuals are taught how to evaluate their own responses to these modalities.

Holistic nurses prescribe as legally authorized. They instruct individuals regarding drug, herbal, and homeopathic regimens and, importantly, the side effects and interactions of these therapies. They consult, collaborate, and refer, as necessary, to both conventional allopathic providers and to holistic practitioners. They provide information and counseling to people about alternative, complementary, integrative, and conventional healthcare practices. Very importantly, holistic nurses facilitate negotiation of services as they guide individuals and families between conventional Western medical and complementary/alternative/integrative systems. Holistic nurses, in partnership with the individual and others, evaluate the effectiveness of care and any changes in the meaning of the health experience for the individual.

Holistic nurses have taken, and should continue to take, a lead in incorporating a holistic caring perspective and integrating healing strategies into practice and system-wide programs and organizations. More healthcare facilities and settings that want to create integrative care delivery models are recognizing that the most successful models nationally are those that originate from nursing. In fact, more than 42% of hospitals in the 2010 *CAM Survey of Hospitals* indicated that they offer one or more CAM therapies (Health Forum & Samueli Institute, 2010). "It is not a coincidence that many successful integrative programs are directed by nurses" (Mittelman et al., 2010, p. 82), many of whom have assumed leadership positions and are mentoring others in holistic integrative health and healing.

Core Value 3. Holistic Communication, Therapeutic Healing Environment, and Cultural Diversity

Through holistic communication, therapeutic healing environments, and diversity, holistic nurses transform their beliefs into practice, highlighting the *how* of holistic nursing.

The holistic nurse's communication ensures that each individual experiences the presence of the nurse as authentic, caring, compassionate, and sincere. This is more than simply using therapeutic techniques such as responding, reflecting, summarizing, and so on. This is deep listening: listening with all the senses, or, as some say, "listening with the heart and not just the ears." It is done with conscious intention and without preconceptions, busyness, distractions, or analysis. It takes place in the "now" within an atmosphere of shared humanness, human being to human being. Through presence or "being with in the moment," holistic nurses provide each individual with an interpersonal encounter that is experienced as a connection with one who is giving *undivided* attention to that individual's needs and concerns. Using unconditional positive regard, holistic nurses convey to the individual receiving care the belief in his/her worth and value as a human being, not solely as the recipient of medical and nursing interventions.

The importance of context in understanding the person's health experience is always recognized. Space and time are allowed for exploration. Each person's health encounter is truly seen as unique and the holistic nurse recognizes that it may be contrary to conventional knowledge and treatments. Therefore, the holistic nurse must be comfortable with ambiguity, paradox, and uncertainty. This requires a perspective that the nurse is not "the expert" regarding another person's health/illness experience, but is actually a "learner."

Holistic nurses have a knowledge base of the use and meanings of symbolic language and use interventions such as imagery, creation of sacred space and personal rituals, dream exploration, narrative, story, journaling, and aesthetic therapies such as music, visual arts, and dance. They encourage and support others in the use of prayer, meditation, and/or other spiritual and symbolic practices for healing purposes.

A cornerstone of holistic nursing practice is assisting individuals to find meaning in their experience. Regardless of their health/illness conditions, the meaning that individuals ascribe to their situations can influence their response to those situations. Holistic nurses attend to the subjective world of the individual. They consider meanings such as the person's concerns in relation to health, family relationships, independence, employment, and economics, as well as to deeper meanings related to the person's purpose in life. Regardless of the technology or treatment, holistic nurses address the human spirit as a major force in healing. The person's perception of meaning is related to all factors in health-wellness-disease-illness.

Holistic nurses realize that suffering, illness, and disease are natural components of the human condition and have the potential to teach about oneself, one's relationships, and the universe. Every experience is valued for its meaning and lesson.

Holistic nurses have a particular obligation to create a therapeutic healing environment that values holism, caring, social support, and integration of conventional and CAM approaches to healing. They seek to create caring cultures and environments or habitats for healing where individuals—whether clients, families, or staff—feel connected, supported, and respected. Holistic nurses shape the physical environment (e.g., light, fresh air, pleasant sounds or quiet, neatness and order, healing smells, earth elements) and, as Nightingale stated, put the person in the best condition for nature to act upon him or her. A particular perspective of holistic nursing is the nurse as the "healing environment" and an instrument of healing. What the nurse brings to a situation can change the environment. The nurse uses his/her consciousness, voice, touch—whole being—for healing. By patterning her/his own energy field to be unified, harmonious, peaceful, ordered, and calm, the nurse provides the client the opportunity within the mutual person–environment process to tune into and resonate with the nurse's healing frequency. The holistic nurse provides a relationship-focused environment, creating through presence and intention sacred space where others can feel safe, unfold, and explore the dimensions of self in healing.

Given their awareness of the dynamic interplay of internal, interpersonal, behavioral, and physical environments, holistic nurses develop self-awareness of personal practices supporting their inner healing environment and integrate professional strategies to improve the healing of the external environment. They recognize that as a microcosm of the macrocosm, their personal health and the health of the planet are intricately intertwined. Thus, they engage in activities that create healing environments for self, home, workplace, and community, and they take risks to challenge current systems and create healthier environments locally and globally (Luck & Keegan, 2013).

Holistic nurses have been integral in the movement to transform organizational cultures to create optimal healing environments. Such institutions as Abbott Northwestern Hospital in Minneapolis, Planetree International, Woodwinds in Minnesota, Beth Israel in New York, Benson Henry Institute in Massachusetts, St. Charles Medical Center in Oregon, Scripts Center for Integrative Medicine in California, Watson Caritas Units, and the Veterans Administration Optimal Healing Initiative are only a few of the institutions nationally in which holistic nurses have provided leadership in transforming organizations to authentic healing healthcare systems (Mittelman et al., 2010). Holistic nurses play a key role "in facilitating this level of change [true healing healthcare] in existing systems and in revisioning/re-creating hospitals and clinics, wellness centers and hospices as *Habitats for Healing*, i.e. optimal healing environments in which nurses thrive and patients heal" (Quinn, 2013).

Of particular importance to holistic nurses is the human connection with the ecology. They actively participate in building an ecosystem that sustains the well-being of all life. This includes raising the public's consciousness about global and environmental issues and stressors that affect not only the health of people, but also the health of the planet. Eco caring is as important as human caring.

Culture, beliefs, and values are an inherent component of a holistic approach. Concepts of health and healing are based in culture and often influence people's actions in promoting, maintaining, and restoring health.

Culture also may provide an understanding of a person's concept of the illness or disease and appropriate treatment. Holistic nurses possess knowledge and understanding of numerous cultural traditions and healthcare practices from various racial, ethnic, and social backgrounds. However, holistic nurses honor individuals' unique understanding and articulation of their own cultural values, beliefs, and health practices rather than relying on stereotypical cultural classifications and descriptions. These understandings are then used to provide culturally competent care that corresponds with the beliefs, values, traditions, and health practices of individuals and families. Holistic nurses ask individuals, "What do I need to know about you culturally in caring for you?"

Holistic healing is a collaborative approach. Holistic nurses take an active role in trying to remove the political and financial barriers to the inclusion of holistic care in the healthcare system. They advocate to influence social and political policy for the betterment of humankind.

Core Value 4. Holistic Education and Research

Holistic nursing is further realized through education and research.

Holistic nurses possess an understanding of a wide range of cultural norms and healthcare practices/beliefs/values concerning individuals, families, groups, and communities from varied racial, ethnic, spiritual, and social backgrounds. This rich knowledge base reflects their formal academic and continuing education preparation and also includes a wide diversity of practices and modalities outside of conventional allopathic medicine. Because of this preparation, holistic nurses serve as both educators and advocates and have a significant impact on people's understanding of healthcare options, alternatives, and choices.

Additionally, holistic nurses, through comprehensive health counseling, motivational interviewing, and coaching, provide much-needed information to individuals on health promotion and disease prevention, on topics such as healthy lifestyles, risk-reducing behaviors, preventive self-care, stress management, living with changes secondary to illness and treatment, and opportunities to enhance well-being.

Holistic nurses value all the ways of knowing and learning. They assess health literacy, individualize learning and teaching, and appreciate that science, intuition, reflection, introspection, creativity, aesthetics, and culture produce different bodies of knowledge and perspectives. They help others to know themselves and access their own inner wisdom to enhance growth, wholeness, and well-being and experience personal transformation in healing.

Holistic nurses often guide individuals and families in their healthcare decisions, especially regarding conventional allopathic and complementary alternative interventions. Therefore, they must be knowledgeable about the best evidence available for both conventional and alternative/integrative therapies. In addition to developing evidence-based/informed practice using research, practice guidelines, and expertise, holistic nurses strongly consider the person's values and healthcare actions, customs, behaviors, and beliefs in practice decisions.

Holistic nurse educators, through the American Holistic Nurses Association, had a significant influence in the revision of the *Essentials of Baccalaureate Education for Professional Nursing Practice* (American Association of Colleges of Nursing [AACN], 2008). The new *Essentials* now include language on preparing the baccalaureate generalist graduate to practice from a holistic, caring framework; engage in self-care; develop an understanding of complementary and alternative modalities; and incorporate patient teaching and health promotion, spirituality, and caring, healing techniques into practice.

Holistic nurses look at alternative philosophies of science and research methods that are compatible with investigations of humanistic and holistic occurrences; that explore the context in which phenomena occur and the meaning of patterns that evolve; that study people and human/social problems holistically; and that take into consideration the interactive nature of body, mind, emotion, energy, spirit, and environment. In order to understand wholeness, healing, and the person–environment dynamic more fully, holistic nurses use all ways of knowing, including empiric, ethical, aesthetic, personal, narrative, transpersonal, embedded, sociopolitical, and unknowing. Holistic nurses engage in praxis or reflection in action, understanding that knowledge, theory, research, evidence, and practice each inform the others. Research approaches and methods can include quantitative, qualitative, triangulated or mixed method, meta-analysis, translational, reflective, appreciative, transpersonal, and whole person/whole system.

To be holistic nursing research, however, the theoretical basis and interpretation of results must be within the context of holism (AHNA, 2009). Holistic nurses conduct and evaluate research in diverse areas such as:

- Outcome measures of various holistic therapies (e.g., Therapeutic Touch, prayer, aromatherapy, imagery, etc.)

- Instrument development to measure holistic phenomena; caring behaviors and dimensions; spirituality; self-transcendence; cultural competence; intuition; presence; mindfulness; etc.

- Client responses to holistic interventions in health/illness/wellness

- Explorations of clients' lived experiences with various health/illness/life phenomena

- Health decision-making

- Health and wellness promotion and illness prevention

- Theory development in healing, wholeness, caring, intentionality, well-being, compassion, social and cultural constructions, empowerment, etc.

- Healing relationships and healing environments

- Teaching and evaluation of holism

Advancements in holistic nursing knowledge development and application in research, education, and practice continue to be disseminated through peer-reviewed journals such as the *Journal of Holistic Nursing (JHN)*, *Holistic Nursing Practice*, and *International Journal of Human Caring*.

Core Value 5. Holistic Nurse Self-Reflection and Self-Care

Self-reflection and self-care, as well as personal awareness of and continuous focus on being an instrument of healing, are significant requirements for holistic nurses.

Self-reflection is both a self-care strategy and a professional practice integrating critical thinking of the mind and compassion of the heart (Levin & Reich, 2013). Holistic nurses reflect in action to become aware of values, beliefs, feelings, sensations, perceptions, and judgments that may affect their actions, and reflect on their experience to obtain insight for future practice. Self-reflection allows one to know oneself more fully in order to become more authentic and mindful.

Holistic nurses value themselves and mobilize the necessary resources to care for themselves. They endeavor to integrate self-awareness, self-care, self-healing, and self-responsibility into their lives by incorporating practices such as self-assessment, meditation, yoga, good nutrition, energy therapies, movement, creative expression (e.g., art, music), support, and lifelong learning. Holistic nurses honor their unique patterns and the development of the body, the psychological-social-cultural self, the intellectual self, and the spiritual self. Nurses cannot facilitate healing within others unless they are in the process of healing themselves. Through continuing education, practice, and self-work, holistic nurses develop the skills of authentic and deep self-reflection and introspection needed to understand themselves and their journey. It is recognized as a lifelong process.

Holistic nurses strive to achieve harmony/balance in their own lives and to assist others to do the same. They create healing environments for themselves by attending to their own well-being, letting go of self-destructive behaviors and attitudes, and practicing centering and stress-reduction techniques. By doing this, holistic nurses serve as role models to others, be they clients, colleagues, or personal contacts.

Holistic nurses have played instrumental roles in creating and implementing self-care programs to increase health and well-being and actualize health potential and promotion for patients, clients/families, communities, healthcare staff, and nurses themselves. Holistic nurses now conduct numerous holistic assessment and intervention classes, courses, and coaching programs in healthcare, worksite, community, and educational and staff development settings. These classes and programs may focus on body/physical, emotional/mental, social/spiritual wellness; stress management; self-care strategies, vibrant living; health promotion and disease prevention activities and lifestyle; environmental health; and healing/caring cultures. Recent research on the effects of holistic self-care programs for nurses and nursing students demonstrates that such programs foster good health behaviors; resilience; improved nurse–patient communication, care, and satisfaction; and improved work environments; and may help sustain the nursing profession.

Settings for Holistic Nursing Practice

Holistic nurses practice in numerous settings. These include, but are not limited to, ambulatory outpatient settings; acute care hospitals; long-term and extended care facilities, nursing homes, and assisted-living facilities; home care; complementary/alternative/integrative care centers; women's health and birthing centers; hospice and palliative care; psychiatric/mental health facilities; private practitioner offices; schools; rehabilitation centers; religious parishes; community health and primary care centers; student and employee health clinics; managed care organizations; independent self-employed private practice; telehealth and cyber care services; correctional facilities; international and travel nursing; military; professional nursing and healthcare organizations; informatics; administration; staff development; and universities and colleges.

Holistic nursing practice also occurs when there is a request for consultation or when holistic nurses advocate for care that promotes health and prevents disease, illness, or disability for individuals, communities, or the environment. For example, a holistic nurse may choose not to work in a clinical care setting, but to provide consultation regarding self-care or stress management to nurses in that setting. Holistic nurses may also practice in preoperative and recovery rooms; for instance, instituting a "Prepare for Surgery" program that teaches individuals having surgery meditation and positive affirmation techniques for use both before and after surgery, while incorporating a homeopathic regimen for trauma and cell healing. Or a holistic nurse may specialize in forensics, focusing on the legal parameters of alternative/complementary/integrative modalities in nursing practice and health care. Employment or voluntary participation of holistic nurses can also influence civic activities and the regulatory and legislative arena at the local, state, national, or international level.

As holistic nursing focuses on wellness, wholeness, and development of the whole person, holistic nurses also practice in health enhancement settings such as spas, gyms, and wellness centers. With all populations and in any setting, holistic nurses empower individuals, families, and groups by teaching them self-care practices for a healthier lifestyle. Additionally, there are numerous entrepreneurial possibilities for holistic nurses to develop integrative care programs in hospitals, home care, primary care practices, occupational and school settings, and the community.

With the explosion of social media during the past decade, holistic nurses have a unique opportunity to inform and educate, both locally and globally, about holistic health and wellness; develop supportive networks; and broadly introduce and influence a more holistic, caring approach to the well-being of all people.

Because holistic nursing is a worldview—a way of "being" in the world and not just a modality—holistic nurses can practice in any setting, anywhere, and with individuals throughout the lifespan. As the public increasingly requests CAM/integrative services and a comprehensive humanistic emphasis on the whole person, holistic nurses will be increasingly in demand and practice in a wider array of settings. Holistic nursing takes place wherever healing occurs.

Educational Preparation for Holistic Nursing Practice

A registered nurse may prepare for the specialty of holistic nursing in a variety of ways. Educational offerings range from undergraduate and graduate courses and programs to continuing education programs with extensive contact hours.

Holistic nurses are registered nurses who are educationally prepared for practice from an approved school of nursing and are licensed to practice in their individual state, commonwealth, or territory. The holistic registered nurse's experience, education, knowledge, and abilities establish the level of competence. Regardless of the level of practice, all holistic nurses integrate the previously identified five core values. This document identifies the scope of practice of holistic nursing and the specific standards and associated competencies of holistic nurses at both the basic and advanced levels.

Basic Practice Level

The education of all nursing students preparing for RN licensure includes basic content on physiological, psychological, emotional, and some spiritual processes with populations across the lifespan, as well as conventional nursing care interventions within each of these domains. Additionally, basic nursing education incorporates experiences in a variety of clinical/practice settings ranging from acute care to community. However, the educational focus is most frequently on "specialties," often emanating from the biomedical disease model with a cure orientation.

In holistic nursing, the individual across the lifespan is viewed in context as an integrated body-mind-emotion-social-spirit-energetic totality, with the emphasis on wholeness, well-being, health promotion, and healing using both conventional and complementary/alternative/integrative practices. Because of the lack of intentional focus on integration, unity, and healing, the educational exposure of most nursing students is not adequate preparation for the specialty role of a holistic nurse.

Currently, there are 10 undergraduate programs in the United States endorsed by the American Holistic Nurses Certification Corporation that prepare undergraduate students in holistic nursing. Additionally, many schools of nursing offer both graduate and undergraduate courses in "Holistic Nursing." Although there are a number of reports in the literature documenting the inclusion of integrative modalities and holistic health and healing in nursing educational programs, the only formal survey to date to discuss the incorporation of holistic nursing practices and CAM into curricula of schools of nursing in the United States was conducted by Fenton and Morris in 2003. This survey indicated that almost 60% ($n = 74$) of the responding schools (sample $n = 125$ schools) had a definition of holistic nursing in their curricula and were familiar with *Holistic Nursing Core Curriculum*. The majority of the sample (84.8%, $n = 106$) included at least one complementary/alternative/integrative modality (e.g., visualization, relaxation, herbal preparations, prayer/meditation) in their curricula. Twenty-six (21%) schools had faculty who were certified in holistic nursing.

Increasingly, schools of nursing are embracing holistic nursing practices and complementary/alternative/integrative modalities and adding them to the curriculum, partly in response to consumer use of CAM and consumer demand for health professionals who are knowledgeable about holistic practices. The new *Essentials of Baccalaureate Education for Professional Nursing Practice* (AACN, 2008) now include language on preparing the baccalaureate generalist graduate to practice from a holistic, caring framework; engage in self-care; develop an understanding of complementary and alternative modalities; and incorporate patient teaching and health promotion, spirituality, and caring, healing techniques into practice. This acknowledges that nursing recognizes the importance of healing principles and practices in health care and the need for nurses to learn them in the educational process.

Advanced Practice Level

As with the basic level, there are a variety of ways (both academic and professional development) in which registered nurses can acquire the additional specialized knowledge and skills that prepare them for advanced holistic nursing practice. These nurses are expected to hold a master's or doctoral degree and demonstrate a greater depth and scope of knowledge, a greater integration of information, increased complexity of skills and interventions, and notable role autonomy. They provide leadership in practice, teaching, research, consultation, management, advocacy, and/or policy formation in advancing holistic nursing to improve the holistic health of people.

In line with the 2008 *Consensus Model for APRN Regulation* (APRN Consensus Work Group & National Council of State Boards of Nursing [NCSBN] APRN Advisory Committee, 2008), beginning in 2015, APRN specialty practice and education in holistic nursing will build upon and will be in addition to education and preparation in one of the four APRN roles and one of the six population foci. "Education programs preparing individuals with additional knowledge in a specialty [holistic nursing], *if used for entry into advanced practice registered nursing and for regulatory purposes*, must also prepare individuals in one of the four nationally recognized APRN roles, and in one of the six population foci. Individuals must be recognized and credentialed in one of the four APRN roles within at least one population [focus]. However, if not intended for entry-level preparation in one of the four roles/population foci and not for regulatory purposes, education programs, using a variety of formats and methodologies, may provide licensed APRNs with the additional knowledge, skills, and abilities to become professionally certified in the specialty area of APRN practice [holistic nursing]" (APRN Consensus Work Group & NCSBN, 2008).

This is a significant transition period for graduate programs in holistic nursing, and schools are exploring various options for curriculum change to meet new criteria. Presently five graduate programs in the United States that prepare master's students with a specialty in holistic nursing are endorsed by the AHNCC. Other graduate nursing programs have courses in holistic or complementary/alternative/integrative practices. Current advanced practice registered nurses (certified nurse practitioners, clinical nurse specialists, certified nurse-midwives, certified registered nurse anesthetists) and graduate-prepared nurse educators, administrators, Doctors of Nursing Practice, and other graduate-prepared nurses in such areas as public health, forensics, and case management are increasingly gaining specialized knowledge that prepares them as holistic nurses through post-master's degree programs, continuing education offerings, and certificate programs.

Continuing Education for Basic and Advanced Practice Levels

The American Holistic Nurses Association is a provider and approver of continuing education, recognized by the American Nurses Credentialing Center (ANCC). Continuing education programs, workshops, and lectures on holistic nursing, healing, CAM, and self-development have been popular nationwide, with AHNA or other bodies granting continuing education units.

AHNA also endorses certificate programs in specific areas. These include Spirituality, Health, and Healing; Integrative Reflexology; Clinical Aromatherapy for Health Professionals; Integrative Aromatherapy; Healing Touch Program; Healing Touch; Holistic Coaching Training Program; Holistic Stress Management Instructor Certification; RN Patient Advocate; Holistic and Integrative Health; Integrative Healing Arts Program; the Great River Craniosacral Therapy Training Program; and Whole Health Education. AHNA approves continuing education offerings in holistic nursing, as well as offering the AHNA home study course "Foundations of Holistic Nursing"; an Introduction to Holistic Nursing module; three Geriatric Care modules; continuing nursing education activities through the *Journal of Holistic Nursing (JHN)*; continuing education online (CNE Online); and workshops at the annual AHNA conference. Additionally, AHNA now offers a monthly webinar series on a variety of holistic and CAM topics.

Other programs in distinct therapies (such as acupuncture, Reiki, homeopathy, massage, imagery, healing arts, holistic health, Oriental medicine, nutrition, Ayurveda, Therapeutic Touch, Healing Touch, herbology, chiropractic, etc.) are offered nationally as degrees, certificates, or continuing education programs by centers, specialty organizations, professional associations, and schools.

Certification in Holistic Nursing

In 1992, a four-phase AHNA Certificate Program in Holistic Nursing began. On completion of the program, a nurse was awarded a certificate in holistic nursing. In 1994, the AHNA Leadership Council appointed an AHNA Task Force Committee to explore the development of holistic nursing certification through a national certification examination.

The AHNA Leadership Council appointed an AHNA Certification Committee to serve as the governing body to oversee the process of certification of holistic nurses by examination until a separate certification corporation was established. In 1997, the AHNA Certification Board established a separate 501(c)(6) organization, the American Holistic Nurses Certification Corporation (AHNCC), to act as the credentialing body for the holistic nursing certification examination. The AHNCC now has six directors who are voting members, and one nonvoting member. All the directors who serve on the AHNCC have been chosen for their skill in and knowledge of the process of certification. There is a public member who is not a registered nurse.

The AHNCC is an autonomous body with administrative independence in matters pertaining to specialty certification. The AHNCC maintains a collaborative relationship with, but is not involved in, the continuing education, endorsement, or accreditation activities of AHNA.

The AHNCC defines *certification* as a qualifying process that a nongovernmental authority uses to grant recognition to an individual who has met specified qualifications and competencies in a defined area of practice. Based on predetermined standards of professional practice, a registered nurse validates her/his qualifications and specialized clinical knowledge for practice by seeking the credential conferred by such an authority. In relation to holistic nursing certification, the nurse must demonstrate competencies of specialized nursing practice encompassing holism.

The purposes of national certification are to establish the minimum knowledge and competencies for holistic nursing practice, to assure the public that the certified nurse has completed all eligibility requirements and earned a credential verifying that he/she has achieved the level of knowledge and competency required for practice of holistic nursing, and to recognize nurses who have met those standards. The AHNCC offers four certifications: *Holistic Nurse, Board Certified* (HN-BC), which requires a minimum of a diploma or associate degree in nursing from an accredited school; *Holistic Baccalaureate Nurse, Board Certified* (HNB-BC), which requires a baccalaureate degree in nursing from an institution regionally accredited by the Association of Schools and Colleges (ASC); and *Advanced Holistic Nurse, Board Certified* (AHN-BC), and *Advanced Practice Holistic Nurse Certification examination* (APHN-BC, APRN), which require a master's degree in nursing from an institution regionally accredited by ASC. At the advanced level, holistic nursing specialty competencies will continue to be assessed separately through the certification process of AHNCC. However, AHNCC is planning to explore what changes in the Advanced Holistic Nurse competencies would be necessary to meet the APRN requirements for certification defined by the 2008 *Consensus Model for APRN Regulation*.

Eligibility criteria for all candidates include: an unrestricted and current U.S. RN license from an academically accredited school of nursing; active practice as a holistic nurse for a minimum of one year full-time or 2,000 hours within the past five years part-time; and completion of a minimum of 48 contact hours of continuing education in holistic nursing within a two-year period preceding application. The application criteria and process can be found at www.ahncc .org/home/certificationprocess.

The process for beginning certification includes a formal review of an applicant's application documenting the practice of holistic nursing (RN licensure, academic credentials, holistic nursing experience, continuing education), a self-reflection assessment, and a quantitative certification exam. Recertification for all three levels is completed by documentation of contact hours in holistic nursing.

Further, AHNCC provides endorsement for university-based undergraduate and graduate nursing programs whose curricula meet the holistic nursing standards detailed in this book. Graduates from "Endorsed Programs" are eligible for waiver of postgraduate practice and continuing education requirements. Those currently in process are also eligible for waiver of the self-reflective assessment requirement.

Continued Commitment to the Profession

Each holistic nurse must educate other nurses, healthcare providers, other disciplines, and the public about the role, value, and benefits of holistic nursing, whether it be in direct practice, education, management, or research. Holistic nurses articulate the ideas underpinning the holistic paradigm and the philosophy of the caring–healing model. Jean Watson reminds us that society and the public are searching for something deeper in terms of realizing self-care, self-knowledge, and self-healing potentials. Nurses need to acknowledge the human aspects of practice, attending to people and their experience rather than just focusing on the medical orientation and disease. She concludes that "nurses have a covenant with the public to sustain caring. It is our collective responsibility to transform caring practices into the framework that identifies and gives distinction to nursing as a profession" (Watson, 2005, p. 12).

Holistic nurses are committed to continuous, lifelong learning and personal growth for themselves and others. As role models, they engage in self-assessment and commit to practicing self-care to enhance their physical, psychological, intellectual, social, and spiritual well-being.

Holistic nurses promote the advancement of the profession and holistic nursing by participating in professional and community organizations, and by writing, publishing, and speaking to professional and lay or public audiences. By engaging in local, state, national, and international forums, they strive to increase the awareness of holistic health issues and the development of holistic care models.

Holistic nurses are particularly attentive to their role as advocates for both people and the environment. They seek to understand the political, social, ethnic, organizational, financial, and discriminatory barriers to holistic care for individuals, population groups, and communities. Holistic nurses work to eliminate these barriers, particularly for the repressed and underserved. They respect and honor people's dignity and freedom to choose among existing alternatives. Holistic nurses assist and empower people to develop skills for self-advocacy and make educated choices about their lives.

Holistic nurses engage in activities that respect, nurture, and enhance humans' integral relationship with the earth, contributing to creating an ecosystem that supports the well-being of all life. Acting as teachers, leaders, collaborators, and consultants, they evaluate global health issues and environmental safety, and assist in reducing or eliminating the effects of environmental hazards on the health or welfare of individuals, groups, and communities.

Care of Older Adults in Holistic Nursing

Holistic nursing care is provided to people of all ages across the entire continuum of care, from health promotion and wellness care to acute illness care. Many of the health promotion and wellness activities and therapies addressed in the following discussion are also incorporated into holistic nursing care for infants, children, adolescents, and adults, in order to promote health and wellness and prevent development of, effectively manage, or reduce the impact of chronic disease or illness.

Holistic nursing recognizes that older adults represent the predominant population in the healthcare delivery system, and constitute a unique population who can benefit greatly from holistic nursing services. The older population—persons 65 years or older—numbered 39.6 million in 2009. They represented 12.9% of the U.S. population, or about one in every eight Americans. By 2030, there will be about 72.1 million older persons, more than twice their number in 2000. People aged 65 or more represented 12.4% of the population in the year 2000, but are expected to constitute 19% of the population by 2030 (Administration on Aging, 2011).

Aging is a multidimensional experience that encompasses the interrelatedness of the body-mind-emotion-energy-spirit-environment totality. It includes physical, sensory, affective, cognitive, behavioral, sociocultural, and spiritual elements. Because aging is a holistic experience, the older adult must be approached in an individualized and comprehensive manner.

As a result of advances in health care during the past century, nurses are caring less frequently for people dying from the infections and accidents that were major sources of mortality at the turn of the century. Today nurses are often caring for older adults with chronic illnesses, which are a significant source of morbidity and mortality. Older adults dying of infectious processes tend to do so as a result of complications of a chronic illness or debilitation. These chronic conditions contribute significantly to increased healthcare costs. Most of these leading causes of disability and death in the United States are modifiable, and in some instances are preventable. In addition, despite an increased incidence of disease and disability, poor health is not an inevitable consequence of aging. Adopting healthy lifestyles—getting regular physical exercise, having social support, maintaining a healthy diet, avoiding tobacco and substance use, and receiving regular healthcare screeningss (e.g., for breast, cervical, and colorectal cancers, for diabetes, and for depression)—can dramatically reduce a person's risk of chronic illnesses.

Not only do a majority of elders experience a chronic condition, but most also have to live with and manage several chronic conditions concurrently. Adopting better lifestyle habits, in conjunction with many of the complementary modalities available to older adults, holds tremendous potential for improving quality of life for older adults, as well as decreasing the co-morbidities (e.g., immobility, pain, dementia) associated with chronic illnesses. Many chronic conditions could be aided by a holistic approach and a variety of complementary/alternative/integrative therapies.

A survey of consumer use of CAM by the American Association of Retired Persons (AARP) and the National Center for Complementary and Alternative Medicine (NCCAM) found that people 50 years of age and older tend to be high users of complementary and alternative medicine (AARP/NCCAM, 2011). More than one-half (53%) of people 50 years and older reported using CAM at some point in their lives, and nearly as many (47%) reported using it in the past 12 months. The most common reasons for using CAM were to prevent illness or for overall wellness (77%), to reduce pain or treat painful conditions (73%), to treat a specific health condition (59%), or to supplement conventional medicine (53%).

Most users of CAM therapies do so without the knowledge or guidance of any healthcare professional. This certainly can pose a risk in geriatric care, in that older adults may be:

- Self-diagnosing and self-treating with CAM products and therapies that could delay the diagnosis and perhaps more appropriate treatment for a health condition

- Unknowingly subjecting themselves to complications associated with interactions or adverse reactions to CAM therapies

- Wasting limited funds on CAM products and services that are ineffective for their specific conditions

Nurses can make a critical difference in assuring that older adults receive maximum benefit at minimum risk as they integrate CAM and conventional therapies. Older adults benefit from use of holistic complementary/alternative/integrative therapies because:

- Holistic therapies build on the body's capabilities and are aimed at strengthening the body's own defenses and healing abilities so that it can do for itself. Strengthened and healthy defenses offer benefits that exceed symptom management, for older adults and all persons.

- Total health state is considered and a balanced lifestyle is promoted to control existing health problems, prevent new problems, and enhance general health state.

- Holistic therapies view the person holistically, realizing that people are complex combinations of unique bodies, minds, emotion, and spirits. CAM considers this interconnectedness as it assesses and addresses the physical, mental, emotional, environmental, and spiritual aspects of the person.

- Healing practices are tailored to the individual. This is especially true for older adults, each of whom is the product of an individualized aging process. Whole-person practices offer customized healing measures.

- Holistic therapies empower older adults and encourage self-care. People are taught about self-care practices, guided in using them, and assisted in exploring obstacles that could stand in the way of doing so. Older adults are empowered when they are encouraged to take maximum responsibility for their own care. Also, family members and caregivers can be taught simple holistic techniques to use with their loved ones and themselves, thereby empowering the caregivers/family to participate in the older adult's care and reduce their own stress.

- The older adult is honored by receiving the attention he or she needs. The abbreviated office visit, common in conventional practice, causes many older persons to feel that they must be selective in what they tell their healthcare provider. As a result, questions, emotional problems, socioeconomic concerns, and spiritual issues that affect health may not be shared. In contrast, holistic practitioners are more likely to spend time learning about the total person and addressing needs holistically.

- Most holistic therapies are safer and gentler than conventional therapies. A variety of age-related changes, combined with the high volume and nature of medications used, make drugs riskier for older adults. Although there are conditions for which drugs provide remarkable benefit, there are other conditions that can be better managed and improved through lower-risk CAM approaches.

(Adapted from Eliopolous, 2009)

With the many benefits that can be derived from using CAM and a holistic approach, holistic nurses can best assist older adults by helping them to integrate CAM with conventional therapies. This requires that nurses understand the intended and safe use of various CAM therapies, educate older adults in appropriate CAM use, and prepare themselves to offer selected CAM therapies as part of their practice.

As part of its continued commitment to improve the quality of health care for older adults and to advance geriatric competence in holistic nursing practice, AHNA offers a series of continuing education modules on topics related to geriatric nursing. These modules were developed through a Nurse Competency in Aging grant from ANA and the John A. Hartford Foundation Institute for Geriatric Nursing, New York University. In 2011, AHNA endorsed the Specialty Nurses Association *Global Vision Statement on Care of Older Adults* (REASN—Resourcefully Enhancing Aging in Specialty Nursing).

AHNA is disseminating the message that competency in geriatric care is relevant for all nurses, as the demographics of the U.S. population rapidly shift. AHNA is dedicated to making geriatric care an integral part of holistic nursing education. Additionally, AHNA has launched a geriatric nursing resource on its web site with information about caring for older adults as part of holistic nursing practice; visit the Geriatric Holistic Care Resource Center (www.ahna.org/geriatricholistic care).

Current Trends and Issues

(The material in this section has been adapted with permission from Mariano, 2013.)

Health Care in the United States

The National Center for Complementary and Alternative Medicine's *Strategic Plan for 2011–2015* (NCCAM, 2011b) and *Healthy People 2020* (U.S. DHHS, 2010) give priority to enhancing physical and mental health and wellness, preventing disease, and empowering the public to take responsibility for their health. The vision of *Healthy People 2020* is "A society in which all people live long, healthy lives" and its goals are to:

- Attain high-quality, longer lives free of preventable disease, disability, injury, and premature death.

- Achieve health equity, eliminate disparities, and improve the health of all groups.

- Create social and physical environments that promote good health for all.

- Promote quality of life, healthy development, and healthy behaviors across all life stages.

And yet, Western medicine is proving ineffective, wholly or partially, for a significant proportion of common chronic diseases. Furthermore, highly technological health care is too expensive to be universally affordable. In a poll taken in May of 2011, 55% of Americans indicated that the healthcare system has major problems, 50% indicated that the healthcare system needs fundamental changes, and 36% stated that there is so much wrong with the healthcare system that it needs to be completely rebuilt (Public Agenda, 2011).

> *Although medical advances have saved and improved the lives of millions, much of medicine and health care have primarily focused on addressing immediate events of disease and injury, generally neglecting underlying socioeconomic factors, including employment, education, and income and behavioral risk factors. These factors, and others, impact health status, accentuate disparities, and can lead to costly, preventable diseases. Furthermore, the disease-driven approach to medicine and health care has resulted in a fragmented, specialized health system in which care is typically reactive and episodic, as well as often inefficient and impersonal (IOM, 2009, pp. 1–2).*

Chronic diseases—such as heart disease, cancer, hypertension, diabetes, and depression—are the leading causes of death and disability in the United States. Chronic diseases account for 70% of all deaths in the United States (1.7 million deaths each year) and also cause major limitations in daily living for almost 1 out of 10 Americans, or about 25 million people (CDC, 2011).

> *Stress accounts for 80% of all healthcare issues in the United States. Super Stress "is a result of both the changing nature of our daily lives and our choices in lifestyle habits, as well as a series of unfortunate events. Extreme chronic stress . . . has silently become a pandemic that disturbs not only how we perceive our quality of life but also our health and mortality. . . . The APA [American Psychological Association] issued a report on stress, revealing that nearly half of all Americans were experiencing stress at a significantly higher level than the previous year and rated its level as extreme (Lee, 2010).*

Healthcare costs have been rising for several years. Expenditures in the United States for health care surpassed $2.3 trillion in 2008, more than three times the $714 billion spent in 1990. Healthcare expenditures are projected to be $2.7 trillion in 2011 and $4.3 trillion by 2017 (U.S. Census Bureau, 2011). In 2008, U.S. healthcare spending was about $7,681 per resident and accounted for 16.2% of the nation's gross domestic product (GDP); this is among the highest of all industrialized countries. Total healthcare expenditures continue to outpace inflation and the growth in national income (KaiserEdu.org, 2010).

In addition to the rising costs, there is disparity in the numbers of Americans insured for health coverage. The U.S. Census Bureau cites the number of uninsured Americans at 50.7 million, 16.7% of the population, rising from 13.7% in 2000, or almost 1 in 6 U.S. residents (Wolf, 2010). The number of underinsured has grown 60% to 25 million over the past 4 years (HealthCare Problems.org, 2011). With the current healthcare crisis, the high cost of health care, the lack of universal access to health care and the resulting 51 million uninsured Americans, the insurance morass and that industry's control of healthcare spending, the disenchantment and disempowerment of healthcare providers, the frustration of clients, patients, or healthcare consumers, the lack of incentive for practitioners or insurers to foster prevention and health promotion, and the startling lack of measures being taken for quality healthcare outcomes, a new perspective and discussion are needed.

Hyman (2005) suggests that we should focus our national healthcare dialogue on quality-based care rather than simply evidence-based care. Prevention and wellness should be emphasized, including funding and research on comparative approaches to chronic healthcare problems and measurement of the role of complementary/integrative therapies in improving overall healthcare quality and reducing healthcare costs. Kreitzer indicates that nurses are exceedingly well positioned to become the leaders in integrative health, and holistic nursing is at the forefront of this movement through its philosophy, education, practice, research programs, and policy agendas (Mittelman et al., 2010).

Trends in Health Care

The American public increasingly demands health care that is compassionate and respectful, provides options, is economically feasible, and is grounded in holistic ideals. A shift is occurring in health care as people desire to be more actively involved in health decision-making. They have expressed their dissatisfaction with conventional (Western allopathic) medicine and are calling for a care system that encompasses health, quality of life, and a relationship with their providers.

The American public has pursued alternative and complementary care at an ever-increasing rate. In 1993, David Eisenberg and colleagues published a now-classic study indicating that one-third of Americans (61 million people) were using some form of alternative or complementary medicine (Eisenberg et al., 1993). The researchers' ongoing study of the use of alternative/complementary care indicated that the use of such modalities had not only continued, but sharply increased to 42% (83 million Americans). The out-of-pocket dollars the

American public spent on CAM were $12.2 billion, which exceeded the out-of-pocket expenditures for all U.S. hospitalizations and just about equaled the total out-of-pocket expenses for all physician services (Eisenberg et al., 1998).

The most recent survey, the 2007 National Health Interview Survey (Barnes et al., 2008), indicates that 38.3% of adults in the United States aged 18 years and older (almost 4 in 10 adults) and nearly 12% of children aged 17 years and younger (1 in 9 children) used some form of CAM within the previous 12 months. Americans spent $33.9 billion out-of-pocket on CAM during the 12 months prior to the survey. This accounts for approximately 1.5% of total U.S. healthcare expenditures and 11.2% of total out-of-pocket expenditures. More than 38 million adults made an estimated 354.2 million visits to practitioners of CAM (NCCAM, 2009).

People who use CAM approaches seek ways to improve their health and well-being, attempt to relieve symptoms associated with chronic or even terminal illnesses or the side effects of conventional treatments, have a holistic health philosophy or desire a transformational experience that changes their worldview, and want greater control over their health. The majority of individuals using CAM do so to complement conventional care rather than as an alternative to conventional care (Barnes et al., 2008).

According to the *Complementary and Alternative Medicine Survey of Hospitals* conducted by the American Hospital Association and the Samueli Institute, hospitals across the nation are responding to patient demand and integrating CAM services with conventional services. More than 42% of hospitals in the survey indicated that they offer one or more CAM therapies, up from 37% in 2007. Respondents cited patient demand as the primary rationale for offering CAM services (Health Forum & Samueli Institute, 2010).

In the past five to seven years, many conventional healthcare institutions have developed complementary programs, including stress management, energy therapies, healers in the operating rooms, and acupuncture. Programs such as Reiki or Therapeutic Touch for chronic pain, support groups using imagery for breast cancer, and groups espousing meditation for health and wellness are commonly advertised across the United States. Similarly, local pharmacies and health food stores are selling an array of supplements, herbs, homeopathic preparations, vitamins, hormones, and various combinations of these that were not considered marketable five years ago. The number of books, journals, and web sites devoted to complementary, integrative, and holistic healing practices has also dramatically increased.

If safe and effective CAM practices become more available to the general population, special and vulnerable populations should also have access to these services, along with conventional health care. CAM would not be a replacement for conventional health care, but would be some of the available treatment options. In some cases, CAM practices may be an equal or superior option. CAM offers the possibility of a new paradigm of integrated health care that could affect the affordability, accessibility, and delivery of healthcare services for millions of Americans, and holistic nurses are in a key position to offer these services.

Interest in workplace clinics has intensified in recent years (particularly with the newly enacted healthcare reform law), as employers move beyond traditional occupational health and convenience care to offering clinics that provide a full range of wellness, health promotion, and primary care services. Such services may include traditional occupational health; acute care, ranging from low-acuity episodic care to exacerbations of acute chronic conditions; preventive care such as immunizations, lifestyle management, mind–body skills, and screenings; wellness assessments and follow-up, health coaching, and education; and disease management for chronic conditions (Tu et al., 2010/2012). Many of the nation's largest employers are focusing on prevention and disease management by adopting an integrative medicine approach.

The Institute for Alternative Futures, funded by the Kresge Foundation, forecasts that in 2025, prevention will be the major focus of primary care and will be community focused; health will be continually assessed along multiple dimensions that include medical, nutritional, behavioral, psychological, social, spiritual, and environmental conditions. Patient-centered primary care will have evolved to person- and family-centered primary care; the whole person will be the focus of care and individuals will be doing enhanced self-care; all dimensions of health will be addressed by bringing the knowledge of conventional, unconventional, complementary, alternative, traditional, and integrative medicine disciplines to bear across the many different cultural traditions of persons cared for; health care will be available anytime and everywhere. People will have 24/7 access to their relational agent and access by phone, email, or televisit to some human member of the primary care team much of the time (Bezold, 2011).

In a classic report, the White House Commission on CAM Policy (WHCCAMP) *Final Report* (2002) stated that people have come to recognize that a healthy lifestyle can promote wellness and prevent illness and disease, and it recognized that many individuals use CAM modalities to attain this goal. The effectiveness of the healthcare delivery system in the future will depend on its ability to use all approaches and modalities to contribute to a sound base for promoting health. Early interventions that promote the development of good health habits and attitudes could help modify many of the negative behaviors and lifestyle choices that began in adolescence and continue into old age. The recommendations of the report are equally—if not more—important today than when the report was first published. It recommends that:

- More evidence-based teaching about CAM approaches be included in all conventional health professional schools;

- Emphasis be placed on the importance of approaches to prevent disease and promote wellness for long-term health of the American people;

- Teaching of the principles and practices of self-care and lifestyle counseling in professional schools be increased and emphasized, so that health professionals can provide this guidance to their patients in addition to improving their own health; and

- Those in the greatest need, including the chronically ill and those with limited incomes, have access to the most accurate, up-to-date information about which therapies and products may help and which may harm.

Similarly, the Institute of Medicine report titled *Complementary and Alternative Medicine in the United States* (IOM, 2005) recommends that the following receive attention in today's healthcare context:

- Health professionals should take into account a patient's individuality, emotional needs, values, and life issues; implement strategies for reaching those who do not ask for care on their own, including healthcare strategies that support the broader community; and enhance prevention and health promotion.

- Health professions schools (e.g., schools of medicine, nursing, pharmacy, and allied health) should incorporate sufficient information about CAM into the standard curriculum—at the undergraduate, graduate, and postgraduate levels—to enable licensed professions to competently advise patients about CAM.

- Healthcare professional licensing boards and crediting and certifying agencies (for both CAM and conventional medicine) should set competency standards for the appropriate use of both conventional medicine and CAM therapies, consistent with practitioners' scope of practice and standards of referral across health professions.

- A moral commitment of openness to diverse interpretations of health and healing, a commitment to finding innovative ways of obtaining evidence, and an expansion of the knowledge base relevant and appropriate to medical practice.

- Research aimed at answering questions about outcomes of care is crucial to ensuring that healthcare professionals provide evidence-based, comprehensive care that encourages a focus on healing, recognizes the importance of compassion and caring, emphasizes the centrality of relationship-based care, encourages patients to share in decision-making about therapeutic options, and promotes choices in care that can include complementary/alternative/integrative medical therapies when appropriate.

In March of 2010, a comprehensive health reform bill (the 2010 Patient Protection and Affordable Healthcare Act, HR 3590) was signed into law. This law and subsequent legislation focus on provisions to expand health coverage, control health costs, and improve the healthcare delivery system.

Another relatively recent initiative, Wellness Initiative for the Nation (WIN), was created to proactively prevent disease and illness, promote health and productivity, and create well-being and flourishing of the people of the United States (Samueli Institute, 2009). In September of 2010, the Surgeon General convened the National Prevention and Health Promotion Council to create the National Prevention Strategy (U.S. Office of the Surgeon General, 2011). The vision of this strategy is working together (state, local and territorial governments, businesses, health care, education and community faith-based organizations) to improve the health and quality of life for individuals, families, and communities by moving the nation from a focus on sickness and disease to one based on wellness and prevention. The "Strategic Directions" are: Healthy and Safe Communities, Clinical and Community Preventive Services, Empowered People, and Elimination of Health Disparities. The goals are to create community environments that make the healthy choice the easy and affordable choice; to implement effective preventive practices by creating and recognizing communities that support prevention and wellness; to connect prevention-focused health care and community efforts to increase preventive services; to empower and educate individuals to make healthy choices; and to eliminate disparities in traditionally underserved populations.

The Summit on Integrative Medicine and the Health of the Public (IOM, 2009) articulated a number of considerations for healthcare reform:

- The progression of many chronic diseases can be reversed and sometimes even completely healed through lifestyle modifications.

- The environment influences health.

- Improving the primary care and chronic disease care systems is paramount. The new system must focus on prevention and wellness and put the patient at the center of care.

- The reimbursement system must be changed to reward health outcomes rather than procedures.

- For an integrated approach to health care, all healthcare practitioners should be educated in team approaches and the importance of compassionate care that addresses the bio-psycho-social dimensions of health, prevention, and well-being.

- Health care should be supported by evidence, especially evidence for integrative models of care.

- Research must better accommodate multifaceted and interacting factors, including biological predispositions and social and environmental influences.

The preceding driving forces will propel mainstream health care into the future. Access to healthcare providers who possess knowledge and skills in the promotion of healthful living and the integration of holistic/integrative modalities is a critical need for Americans. Holistic nurses are professionals who have knowledge of a wide range of complementary, alternative, and integrative modalities; health promotion and restoration and disease prevention strategies; and relationship-centered, caring ways of healing. They are in a prime position to meet the identified present and future national needs and provide leadership in these trends.

Issues in Holistic Nursing

In December 2006, holistic nursing was officially recognized by the American Nurses Association as a distinct nursing specialty with a defined scope and standards of practice, acknowledging holistic nursing's unique contribution to the health and healing of people and society. This recognition provides holistic nurses with clarity and a foundation for their practice; equally importantly, it gives holistic nursing legitimacy and voice within the nursing profession and credibility in the eyes of the healthcare world and the public.

Nevertheless, a number of issues exist or will emerge in the future for holistic nursing. Acceptance of holistic nursing's influence and input, within both nursing and other disciplines, continues as one of the most pressing matters. Other concerns can be categorized into the areas of education, research, clinical practice, and policy. It is important to note that because holistic nursing (as well as nursing in general) and other disciplines face many of the same issues, an interdisciplinary approach is imperative for success in achieving the desired outcomes.

Education

There are several areas of educational challenge in the holistic arena. With increased use of complementary/alternative/integrative therapies by the American public, both students and faculty need knowledge of these therapies and skill in their use. One urgent priority is the integration of holistic, relationship-centered philosophies and integrative modalities into nursing curricula. Core content appropriate for both basic and advanced practice programs must be identified, and models for integration of both content and practical experiences into existing curricula are necessary. An elective course is not sufficient to impart this knowledge to future practitioners of nursing.

On a positive note, in 2008, AHNA worked with the American Association of Colleges of Nursing in the revision of *Essentials of Baccalaureate Education for Professional Nursing Practice* (AACN, 2008) to incorporate holistic nursing philosophy and practices. These *Essentials* now include language and outcomes on preparing the baccalaureate generalist graduate to: practice from a holistic, caring framework; engage in self-care; develop an understanding of complementary and alternative modalities; and incorporate patient teaching and health promotion, spirituality, and caring, healing techniques into practice. Holistic nurses will need to continue to work with the accrediting bodies of academic degree programs to ensure that this content is included in educational programs.

The 2010 Carnegie Foundation's report, *Educating Nurses: A Call for Radical Transformation* (Benner et al., 2010), notes that the need for better nursing education in nursing, social and natural sciences, humanities, problem-solving, teaching, and interpersonal capacities is even more acute than it was even 10 years ago. It recommends the following:

- Broadening clinical experiences to community health care

- Promoting and supporting students' learning regarding the skills of inquiry and research

- Teaching the ethics of care and responsibility, the ethos of self-care in the profession, and the skills of involvement, clinical reasoning, and reflection

- Teaching strategies for organizational change, organizational development, policy-making, leadership, and improvement of healthcare systems

- Incorporating evidence-based practice and critical reflection

- Assisting students to better understand the patient's context and how they can help patients improve access to and continuity of care

- Teaching relational skills of involvement and caring practices

- Teaching collegial and collaborative skills

The National Educational Dialogue, an outgrowth of the Integrated Healthcare Policy Consortium, sought to identify a set of core values, knowledge, skills, and attitudes necessary for all healthcare professional students. The Task Force on Values, Knowledge, Skills, and Attitudes, chaired by holistic nurse Carla Mariano, identified the following core values to be taught in all health professions schools (Goldblatt et al., 2009):

- Wholeness and healing—interconnectedness of all people and things with healing as an innate capacity of every individual

- Clients/patients/families as the center of practice

- Practice as a combined art and science

- Self-care of the practitioner and commitment to self-reflection, personal growth, and healing

- Interdisciplinary collaboration and integration embracing the breadth and depth of diverse healthcare systems and collaboration with all disciplines, clients, and families

- Responsibility to contribute to the improvement of the community, the environment, health promotion, healthcare access, and the betterment of public health

- Attitudes and behaviors of all participants in health care demonstrating respect for self and others; humility; and authentic, open, courageous communication

There is a definitive need for increased scholarship and financial aid to support training in all of these areas. Faculty development programs also are necessary to support faculty in understanding and integrating holistic philosophy, content, and practices into nursing curricula. This is especially important, as the majority of nursing faculty members do not have extensive knowledge, experience, or skills in holistic or integrative health or therapies.

A major report by the IOM, *The Future of Nursing: Leading Change, Advancing Health* (IOM, 2010), recommends that *nurses should achieve higher levels of education and training through improved educational systems* by increasing the proportion of nurses with a baccalaureate degree to 80% by 2020, doubling the number of nurses with a doctorate by 2020, and ensuring that nurses engage in lifelong learning. Nurses need more education and preparation to adopt new roles quickly in response to rapidly changing healthcare settings and an evolving healthcare system. Competencies are especially needed in community, geriatrics, leadership, health policy, system improvement and change, research and evidence-based practice, and teamwork and collaboration.

To improve the competency of practitioners and the quality of services, holistic and CAM education and training must continue beyond basic and advanced academic education. Continuing education programs at national and regional specialty organizations and conferences may assist in meeting this need. Working with practitioners in other areas of nursing to increase their understanding of the philosophical and theoretical foundations of holistic nursing practices (e.g., consciousness, intention, presence, centering) as well as integrative therapies will be another role of holistic nurses.

Research

Research in the area of holistic nursing will become increasingly important in the future. Three areas of research seem to be widely proposed: whole systems research, exploration of healing relationships, and outcomes of healing interventions, particularly in the areas of health promotion and prevention.

There is a great need for an evidence base to establish the effectiveness and efficacy of complementary/alternative/integrative therapies. One of the formidable tasks for nurses will be to identify and describe outcomes of CAM and holistic therapies, such as healing, well-being, and harmony, and to develop instruments to measure these outcomes. The IOM report on CAM in the United States (IOM, 2005) recommends both qualitative and quantitative research to examine the following:

- The social and cultural dimensions of illness experiences, the processes and preferences of seeking health care, and practitioner–patient interactions

- How often users of CAM, including patients and providers, adhere to treatment instructions and guidelines

- The effects of CAM on wellness and disease prevention

The current mission of the National Center for Complementary and Alternative Medicine, as indicated in the NCCAM Third Strategic Plan, *Exploring the Science of Complementary and Alternative Medicine: 2011–2015* (NCCAM, 2011b), is to develop evidence requiring support across the continuum of basic science (How does the therapy work?), translational research (Can it be studied in people?), efficacy studies (What are the specific effects?), and outcomes and effectiveness research (How well does the CAM practice work in the general population or healthcare settings?).

The 2010 Patient Protection and Affordable Care Act created a Patient-Centered Outcomes Research Institute (http://www.gao.gov/about/hcac/patientcentered_outcomes.html), a nonprofit organization that will act to assist patients, clinicians, purchasers, and policy-makers in making informed health decisions by carrying out research projects that provide quality, relevant evidence on how diseases, disorders, and other health conditions can effectively and appropriately be prevented, diagnosed, treated, monitored, and managed. This patient-centered outcomes research (PCOR) will help people make informed healthcare decisions and allow their voice to be heard in assessing the value of healthcare options.

Presently, most research outcome measures are based on physical or disease symptomatology. However, methodologies must be expanded to capture the wholeness of the individual's experience, because the philosophy of these therapies rests on a paradigm of wholeness.

> *Integrative health care is* derived from lessons integrated across scientific disciplines, and it requires scientific processes that cross domains. *The most important influences on health, for individuals and society, are not the factors at play within any single domain—genetics, behavior, social or economic circumstances, physical environment, health care—but the dynamics and synergies across domains. Research tends to examine these influences in isolation, which can distort interpretation of the results and hinder application of results. The most value will*

come from broader, systems-level approaches and redesign of research strategies and methodologies (IOM, 2009, p. 7).

The *Journal of Alternative and Complementary Medicine* collaborated with the International Society for Complementary Medicine Research (ISCMR) to sponsor a forum on the research issues for *whole* systems. Participants underscored the political and economic challenges of getting research funded and published if researchers look at the practices and processes that typify *whole-person* treatment. What is clear is that whole practices, whole systems, and related research require professional and organizational attention.

Today researchers are being challenged to look at alternative philosophies of science and research methods that are compatible with investigations of humanistic and holistic occurrences. We also need to study phenomena by exploring the context in which they occur and the meaning of patterns that evolve. Also needed are approaches to interventions studies that are more holistic, taking into consideration the interactive *nature of the body-mind-emotion-spirit-environment. Rather than isolating the effects of one part of an intervention, we need more comprehensive interventions and more sensitive instruments that measure the interactive nature of each client's biological, psychological, sociological, emotional, and spiritual patterns. In addition, comprehensive comparative outcome studies are needed to ascertain the usefulness, indications, and contraindications of integrative therapies. Further, researchers must evaluate these interventions for their usefulness in promoting wellness as well as preventing illness (Mariano, 2008).*

Investigations into the concept and nature of the placebo effect are also needed, because one-third of all medical healings are the result of the placebo effect.

Nurses need to get better at securing funding for their holistic research. They need to apply to National Institutes of Health (NIH) centers and institutes other than just the National Institute of Nursing Research for funding, particularly the National Center for Complementary and Alternative Medicine. Going hand-in-hand with this is the need for nurses to be represented on study sections and review panels to educate and convince the biomedical/NIH community about the value of nursing research; the need for models of research focusing on health promotion and disease prevention, wellness, and self-care instead of just the disease model; and the importance of a variety of designs and research methodologies that include qualitative studies, rather than relying solely on randomized controlled trials.

An area of responsibility for advanced practice holistic nurses is the dissemination of their research findings to various media sources (e.g., television, radio, newsprint, Internet) and at nonnursing, interdisciplinary conferences. Publishing in nonnursing journals and serving on editorial boards of nonnursing journals also broadens other disciplines' appreciation for nursing's role in setting the agenda and conducting research in the area of holism and CAM.

Clinical Practice

Clinical care models reflecting holistic assessment, treatment, health, healing, and caring are important in the development of holistic nursing. Implementing holistic and humanistic models in today's healthcare environment will require a paradigm shift for the many providers who subscribe to a disease model of care. Such acceptance poses an enormous challenge. Loretta Ford identified actions that nurse leaders might consider in advancing integrative health (Mittleman et al., 2010, p. 82):

- Create a culture of innovation and involve staff in alternative practices

- Review the institution's philosophy, mission, policies, programs, and practices for opportunities to include alternative therapies

- Influence clinical practice for recognition of patients' personal usage of integrative therapies

- Collaborate and encourage collaboration with other professionals involved in integrative practices

- Support (financially and otherwise) and guide programs of staff recruitment, preparation, and training in integrative care

- Publish nursing programs, studies, and reports on alternative therapy outcomes, issues, and challenges

Given their education and experience, holistic nurses are the logical leaders in integrative care and must advance that position.

Licensure and credentialing pose another challenge for holistic nursing. As complementary/alternative/integrative healthcare has gained national recognition, state boards of nursing have begun to attend to the regulation issues. *The Future of Nursing* report (IOM, 2010) notes that regulations defining scope-of-practice limitations vary widely by state. Some states have kept pace with the evolution of the healthcare system by changing their scope-of-practice regulations, but the majority of state laws lag behind in this regard. As a result, what nurse practitioners are allowed to do once they graduate varies widely; often these constraints are related not to their ability, education or training, or safety concerns but to the political decisions of the state in which they work. The IOM states that *nurses should practice to the full extent of their education and training* and that *scope-of-practice barriers should be removed.* The IOM also recommends the implementation of nurse residency programs.

In 2010, AHNA conducted a preliminary survey to ascertain the number of state boards of nursing that accepted and recognized holistic nursing and/ or had regulations or a nursing practice act that permitted holistic practices. Of the 39 states that responded, 8 states include holistic nursing in their nurse practice act. The findings from a review of actual state practice acts further revealed that 47 of 51 states/territories have some statements or positions that include holistic wording such as *self-care, spirituality, natural therapies,* and/ or specific complementary/alternative/integrative therapies under the scope of practice for nurses in those states.

It will be important in the future to monitor state boards of nursing for evidence of their recognition and support of holistic, integrative nursing practice and requirements that include CAM and holistic modalities. Finally, holistic nursing has the challenge of working with the state boards to incorporate this content into the National Council Licensure Examination, thus ensuring the credibility of this practice knowledge.

Addressing the nursing shortage in this country is crucial to the health of our nation. Nurses often change jobs or leave the profession because of unhumanistic and chaotic work environments and professional and personal burnout. Multiple surveys and studies confirm that the shortage of RNs influences the delivery of health care in the United States and negatively affects patient outcomes. According to the American Hospital Association, the United States is, by all accounts, in the midst of a significant shortage of registered nurses that is projected to last well into the future. Nationally, there is an average vacancy of approximately 116,000 RNs in hospitals. Although shortages of hospital staff nurses have received the greatest amount of national attention, shortages persist in other settings; for example, there are 19,400 RN vacancies in long-term-care settings, bringing the national RN vacancy rate to 8.1% (AACN, 2011). Buerhaus, Auerbach, and Staiger (2009) found that the U.S. nursing shortage is projected to grow to 260,000 RNs by 2025, which would be twice as large as any nursing shortage experienced in this country since the mid-1960s. Because the demand for RNs will increase as large numbers of RNs retire, a large and prolonged shortage of nurses is expected to hit the United States in the latter half of the next decade.

Additionally, there are some distressing statistics: In the United States, 41% of nurses are dissatisfied with their present job. Nationally, nurses give themselves burnout scores of 30–40%, and 17% of nurses are not working in nursing. Moreover, 18% of newly licensed RNs left their first job within one year, 26.2% left within two years, and 37% reported that they felt ready to change jobs (Robert Wood Johnson RN Work Project, 2012).

Research shows that reduction of perceived stress is related to job satisfaction. Holistic nurses, through their knowledge of self-care, resilience, caring cultures, healing environments, and stress management techniques, have an extraordinary opportunity to influence and improve the healthcare milieu, both for healthcare providers and for clients and patients (Mariano, 2007).

Policy

Four major policy issues face holistic nursing in the future: leadership, reimbursement, regulation, and access. The IOM report *The Future of Nursing* (2010) recommends that *nurses should be full partners with physicians and other health professionals in redesigning healthcare in the United States.* Nurses should be prepared and enabled to lead change in all roles—from the bedside to the boardroom—to advance health. Nurses should have a voice in health policy decision-making and be engaged in implementation efforts related to healthcare reform, particularly regarding quality, access, value, and patient-centered care. Holistic nurses must see policy as something they can shape rather than something that happens to or is imposed on them.

Public or private policies regarding coverage and reimbursement for healthcare services play a crucial role in shaping the healthcare system, and will play a crucial role in deciding the future of wellness, health promotion, and CAM in the nation's healthcare system. Often, however, holistic modalities are offered as a supplemental benefit rather than a core or basic benefit, and many third-party payers do not cover such services at all. In the 2010 CAM survey of hospitals (Health Forum & Samueli Institute, 2010), 69% of CAM services were paid for out of pocket by patients. Coverage and reimbursement for most CAM services depend on the provider's ability to legally furnish services within the scope of practice. The legal authority to practice is given by the state in which services are provided.

Reimbursement of advanced practice nurses also depends on appropriate credentials. Holistic nurses will need to work with Medicare and other third-party payers, insurance groups, boards of nursing, healthcare policy-makers, legislators, and other professional nursing organizations to ensure that holistic nurses are appropriately reimbursed for services rendered. Another issue regarding reimbursement is the fact that the effectiveness of CAM is influenced by the holistic focus and integrative skill of the provider. Consequently, reimbursement must be included for the process of holistic and integrative care, not just for providing a specific modality.

There are many barriers to the use of holistic therapies by potential beneficiaries, providing yet another challenge for holistic nurses. Barriers include lack of awareness of the therapies and their benefits, uncertainty about their effectiveness, inability to pay for them, and limited availability of qualified providers. Access is even more difficult for rural populations; uninsured and underinsured populations; special populations, such as racial and ethnic minorities; and vulnerable populations, such as older adults and those with chronic or terminal illnesses. Holistic nurses have a responsibility to educate the public more fully about health promotion, complementary/alternative/integrative modalities, and qualified practitioners and to assist people in making informed choices among the array of healthcare alternatives and individual providers. Holistic nurses also must actively participate in the political arena as leaders in this movement to ensure quality, an increased focus on wellness, and access and affordability for all.

Holistic nurses, by developing theoretical and empirical knowledge as well as caring and healing approaches, will advance holistic nursing practice and education and contribute significantly to the formalization and credibility of this work. They have provided, and will continue to provide, the leadership in the profession in research, the development of educational models, and the integration of a more holistic approach in nursing practice and health care.

Standards of Holistic Nursing Practice

Overarching Philosophical Principles of Holistic Nursing

Holistic nurses express, contribute to, and promote an understanding of the following: a philosophy of nursing that values healing as the desired outcome; the human health experience as a complex, dynamic relationship of health, illness, disease, wellness, and well-being; the scientific foundations of nursing practice; and nursing as an art. The philosophical principles of Holistic Nursing (see pp. 5–8 in this book) are embedded in every Standard of Practice and Standard of Professional Performance.

Standards of Practice for Holistic Nursing

Standard 1. Assessment

The holistic registered nurse collects comprehensive data pertinent to the person's health and/or the situation.

COMPETENCIES

The holistic registered nurse:

- Collects comprehensive data including but not limited to physical, functional, psychosocial, emotional, mental, sexual, cultural, age-related, environmental, spiritual/transpersonal, economic, and energy field assessments in a systematic and ongoing process while honoring the uniqueness of the person.

- Elicits the person's health and cultural practices, values, beliefs, preferences, meanings of health/illness/wellbeing, lifestyle patterns, family issues, and risk behaviors and context.

- Elicits the person's expressed needs, knowledge and understanding of the health care situation, strengths, coping status, and internal and external resources.

- Involves the person, family, significant others, caregivers, and other healthcare providers, as appropriate in holistic data collection.

- Identifies barriers (e.g., psychosocial, literacy, financial, cultural) to effective communication and makes appropriate adaptations.

- Recognizes the impact of personal attitudes, values, and beliefs.

- Assesses family dynamics and impact on healthcare consumer health and wellness.

- Prioritizes data collection based on the person's immediate condition or the anticipated needs of the person or situation.

- Uses appropriate evidence-based assessment techniques, tools, and instruments in collecting pertinent data as a basis for holistic care.

- Synthesizes available data, information, and knowledge relevant to the situation to identify patterns and variances as they relate to the whole person within the life context.

- Applies ethical, legal, and privacy guidelines and policies to the collection, maintenance, use, and dissemination of data and information.

- Recognizes the person as the authority on their own health by honoring their care preferences.

- Documents relevant data in a retrievable format.

- Incorporates various types of knowing, including empiric, ethical, aesthetic, personal, narrative, transpersonal, embedded, socio-political, intuition, and unknowing, when gathering data from the person and validates this knowledge with the person when appropriate.

ADDITIONAL COMPETENCIES FOR THE GRADUATE-LEVEL-PREPARED HOLISTIC NURSE AND THE APRN

The graduate-level-prepared holistic nurse or the advanced practice registered nurse:

- Initiates and interprets diagnostic procedures relevant to the person's current status.

- Assesses the effect of interactions among individuals, family, community, and social systems on health and illness.

- Elicits and uses client narratives to reveal the context and complexity of the health experience.

- Explores the meanings of the symbolic language expressing itself in areas such as dreams, images, symbols, narratives, sensations, and prayers that are a part of the individual's health experience.

Standard 2. Diagnosis

The holistic registered nurse analyzes the assessment data to determine the diagnosis or issues expressed as actual or potential patterns/problems/needs.

COMPETENCIES

The holistic registered nurse:

- Derives the diagnosis or issues from holistic assessment data.

- Assists the person to explore the meaning of the health/disease experience.

- Validates the diagnosis or issues with the person, family/significant other, and other healthcare providers when possible and appropriate.

- Identifies actual or potential risks to the healthcare consumer's health and safety or barriers to health, which may include but are not limited to interpersonal, systematic, or environmental circumstances.

- Uses standardized classification systems and clinical decision support tools, when available, in identifying diagnoses.

- Documents diagnoses or issues in a manner that facilitates determination of the expected outcomes and plan.

ADDITIONAL COMPETENCIES FOR THE GRADUATE-LEVEL-PREPARED HOLISTIC NURSE AND THE APRN

The graduate-level-prepared holistic nurse or the advanced practice registered nurse:

- Systematically compares and contrasts clinical findings with normal and abnormal variations and development events in formulating a differential diagnosis.

- Utilizes complex data and information obtained during interview, examination, and diagnostic procedures in identifying diagnoses.

- Establishes the diagnoses reflecting the level of acuity, severity, and complexity of health patterns/challenges/needs.

- Assists staff in developing and maintaining competency in the diagnostic process.

Standard 3. Outcomes Identification

The holistic registered nurse identifies expected outcomes for a plan individualized to the person or the situation. The holistic nurse values the evolution and the process of healing as it unfolds. This implies that specific unfolding outcomes may not be immediately evident, due to the nonlinear nature of the healing process, so that both expected/anticipated and evolving/emerging outcomes are considered.

COMPETENCIES

The holistic registered nurse:

- Involves the person, family, significant others, and other healthcare providers in formulating expected outcomes when possible and appropriate.

- Derives culturally appropriate expected outcomes from the diagnoses.

- Considers associated risks, benefits, costs, current scientific evidence, trajectory of the condition, and clinical expertise when formulating expected outcomes.

- Defines expected outcomes in terms of the person's values and beliefs, preferences, culture, age, spiritual practices, ethical considerations, environment, or situation.

- Partners with the person to identify realistic goals based on the person's present and potential capabilities and quality of life.

- Assists the person to understand the potential for unfolding outcomes due to the nature of healing.

- Includes a realistic time estimate for attainment of expected outcomes.

- Develops expected outcomes that facilitate continuity of care.

- Modifies expected outcomes according to changes in the status or preference of the person or evaluation of the situation.

- Documents expected outcomes as measurable goals.

- Focuses on the person's attaining, maintaining, or regaining health, healing, well-being, or peaceful dying while honoring all phases of the person's healing process, regardless of expectations or outcomes.

ADDITIONAL COMPETENCIES FOR THE GRADUATE-LEVEL-PREPARED HOLISTIC NURSE AND THE APRN

The graduate-level-prepared holistic nurse or the advanced practice registered nurse:

- Identifies expected outcomes that incorporate scientific evidence and are achievable through implementation of evidence-based practices.

- Identifies expected outcomes that incorporate healthcare consumer satisfaction, the person's understanding and meanings in his/her unique patterns and processes, quality of life, cost, clinical effectiveness, and continuity and consistency among providers.

- Differentiates outcomes that require care process interventions from those that require system-level interventions.

Standard 4. Planning

The holistic registered nurse develops a plan that prescribes strategies and alternatives to attain expected outcomes.

COMPETENCIES

The holistic registered nurse:

- In partnership with the person, family, and others, develops an individualized plan that considers the person's characteristics or situation, including, but not limited to, values, beliefs, knowledge and understanding, spiritual and health practices, preferences, choices, developmental level, coping style, culture and environment, and available technology.

- Establishes the plan priorities with the person, family/significant others, and others, as appropriate.

- Includes strategies in the plan that address each of the identified diagnoses, issues, or opportunities. These may include, but are not limited to, strategies for:

  - Promotion and restoration of health and well-being

  - Prevention of illness, injury, and disease

  - The promotion of comfort and the alleviation of suffering

  - Supportive care for those who are dying

- Includes strategies for health, wholeness, and growth across the lifespan.

- Provides for continuity in the plan.

- Incorporates an implementation pathway or timeline in the plan.

- Considers the economic impact of the plan on the person, family, caregivers, and other affected parties.

- Integrates current scientific evidence, trends, and research.

- Utilizes the plan to provide direction to other members of the health-care team.

- Establishes practice settings and safe space and time for both the nurse and person/family/significant others to explore suggested, potential, and alternative options.

- Defines the plan to reflect current statutes, rules and regulations, and standards.

- Modifies the plan according to ongoing assessment of the healthcare consumer's response and other outcome indicators.

- Documents the plan in a manner that uses standardized language or recognized terminology.

ADDITIONAL COMPETENCIES FOR THE GRADUATE-LEVEL-PREPARED HOLISTIC NURSE AND THE APRN

The graduate-level-prepared holistic nurse or the advanced practice registered nurse:

- Identifies assessment strategies, diagnostic strategies, therapeutic interventions, therapeutic effects, and side effects that reflect current evidence, including data, research, literature, expert clinical knowledge, and the person's experiences.

- Selects or designs, in partnership with the person, strategies to meet the multifaceted holistic needs of complex individuals.

- Supports the use of clinical guidelines for positive outcomes related to the person's healing.

- Includes a synthesis of the person's values, beliefs, preferences, and choices regarding nursing, medical, and complementary/alternative/integrative therapies within the plan.

- Uses linguistic and symbolic language, including but not limited to word associations, dreams, storytelling, and journals, to explore with individuals the possibilities and options.

- Leads the design and development of interprofessional processes to address the identified diagnosis or issue.

- Actively participates in the development and continuous improvement of systems that support the planning process.

Standard 5. Implementation

The holistic registered nurse implements the identified plan in partnership with the person.

COMPETENCIES

The holistic registered nurse:

- Partners with the person, family, significant others, and caregivers as appropriate to implement the plan in a safe, realistic, and timely manner.

- Demonstrates caring behaviors towards healthcare consumers, significant others, and groups of people receiving care.

- Uses self as an instrument of healing.

- Utilizes technology to measure, record, and retrieve healthcare consumer data, implement the nursing process, and enhance nursing practice.

- Utilizes evidence-based interventions and treatments specific to the diagnosis or problem.

- Provides holistic care that addresses the needs of diverse populations across the lifespan.

- Advocates for health care that is sensitive to the needs of the person, with particular emphasis on the needs of diverse populations.

- Applies appropriate knowledge of major health problems and cultural diversity in implementing the plan of care.

- Applies available healthcare technologies to maximize access and optimize outcomes for healthcare consumers.

- Utilizes community resources and systems to implement the plan.

- Collaborates with healthcare providers from diverse backgrounds to implement and integrate the plan.

- Accommodates different styles of communication used by healthcare consumers, families, and healthcare providers.

- Integrates traditional and complementary/alternative/integrative health-care practices as appropriate.

- Implements the plan in a timely manner in accordance with patient safety goals.

- Promotes the person's capacity for the optimal level of participation and problem-solving, honoring the person's choices and unique healing journey.

- Documents implementation and any modifications, including changes or omissions, of the identified plan.

ADDITIONAL COMPETENCIES FOR THE GRADUATE-LEVEL-PREPARED HOLISTIC NURSE AND THE APRN

The graduate-level-prepared holistic nurse or the advanced practice registered nurse:

- Facilitates utilization of systems, organizations, and community resources to implement the plan.

- Supports collaboration with nursing colleagues and other disciplines to implement plans for individuals, families, groups, and communities that integrate biomedical, complementary, and alternative approaches to healing.

- Incorporates new knowledge and strategies to initiate change in nursing care practices if desired outcomes are not achieved.

- Assumes responsibility for safe and efficient implementation of the plan.

- Uses advanced communication skills to promote relationships between nurses and healthcare consumers, to provide a context for open discussion of the person's experiences, and to improve holistic and other healthcare outcomes.

- Actively participates in the development and continuous improvement of systems that support implementation of the plan.

Standard 5A. Coordination of Care

The holistic registered nurse coordinates care delivery.

COMPETENCIES

The holistic registered nurse:

- Organizes the components of the plan.

- Manages the person's care so as to maximize independence and quality of life.

- Assists the person to identify options for alternative care.

- Communicates with the person, family, and system during transitions in care.

- Advocates for the delivery of dignified and humane care by the interprofessional team.

- Documents the coordination of care.

ADDITIONAL COMPETENCIES FOR THE GRADUATE-LEVEL-PREPARED HOLISTIC NURSE AND THE APRN

The graduate-level-prepared holistic nurse or the advanced practice registered nurse:

- Provides leadership in the coordination of interprofessional health care for integrated delivery of person-care services across continuums, settings, and over time.

- Synthesizes data and information to prescribe necessary system and community support measures, including modifications of environment.

Standard 5B. Health Teaching and Health Promotion

The holistic registered nurse employs strategies to promote health/wellness and a safe environment.

COMPETENCIES

The holistic registered nurse:

- Provides health teaching to individuals, families, and significant others or caregivers that enhances the body-mind-emotion-spirit-environment connection by addressing such topics as:

  - Healthy lifestyles

  - Risk-reducing behaviors

  - Developmental needs

  - Activities of daily living

  - Preventive self-care

  - Living with changes secondary to illness and treatment

  - Stress management

  - Opportunities to enhance well-being

- Uses health promotion and health teaching methods appropriate to the situation and the individual's values, beliefs, health practices, age, developmental level, learning needs, readiness and ability to learn, language preference, spirituality, culture, and socioeconomic status.

- Seeks ongoing opportunities for feedback and evaluation of the effectiveness of the strategies used.

- Uses information technologies to communicate health promotion and disease prevention information to the healthcare consumer in a variety of settings.

- Provides appropriate information, including but not limited to intended effects and potential adverse effects of the proposed prescribed agents/ treatments, costs, complementary/alternative/integrative treatments and procedures, and the effects of single and multiple interventions on the person's health and functioning.

■ Creates educational environments that are safe for the exploration necessary for learning.

■ Assists others to access their own inner wisdom that may provide opportunities to enhance and support growth, development, and wholeness.

ADDITIONAL COMPETENCIES FOR THE GRADUATE-LEVEL-PREPARED HOLISTIC NURSE AND THE APRN

The graduate-level-prepared holistic nurse or the advanced practice registered nurse:

■ Synthesizes empirical evidence on risk behaviors, decision-making about life choices, learning theories, behavioral change theories, motivational theories, epidemiology, and other related theories and frameworks when designing holistic health education information and programs.

■ Conducts personalized health teaching and counseling that considers comparative effectiveness research recommendations.

■ Designs health information and education appropriate to the individual's developmental level, learning needs, readiness to learn, and cultural values and beliefs.

■ Evaluates various health information resources, such as the Internet, in the area of practice for accuracy, readability, and comprehensibility, to help the person access quality health information.

■ Engages consumer alliances and advocacy groups, as appropriate, in health teaching and health promotion activities.

■ Provides anticipatory guidance to individuals, families, groups, and communities to promote health and prevent or reduce the risk of health problems.

Standard 5C. Consultation

The graduate-level-prepared holistic nurse or advanced practice registered nurse provides consultation to influence the identified plan, enhance the abilities of others, and effect change.

COMPETENCIES FOR THE GRADUATE-LEVEL-PREPARED HOLISTIC NURSE AND THE APRN

The graduate-level-prepared holistic nurse or the holistic advanced practice registered nurse:

- Synthesizes clinical data, theoretical frameworks, belief/value systems, and evidence when providing consultation.

- Facilitates the effectiveness of a consultation by involving all stakeholders, including the individual, in decision-making and negotiating role responsibilities.

- Communicates consultation recommendations.

Standard 5D. Prescriptive Authority and Treatment

The advanced practice registered nurse uses prescriptive authority, procedures, referrals, treatments, and therapies in accordance with state and federal laws and regulations.

COMPETENCIES FOR THE GRADUATE-LEVEL-PREPARED HOLISTIC NURSE AND THE APRN

The graduate-level-prepared holistic nurse or the advanced practice registered nurse:

- Prescribes evidence-based treatments, therapies, and procedures considering the person's comprehensive healthcare needs and holistic choices.

- Prescribes pharmacologic agents according to current knowledge of pharmacology and physiology.

- Prescribes specific pharmacologic agents and/or treatments based on clinical indicators; the person's status, needs, and age; the results of diagnostic and laboratory tests; and the person's beliefs, values, and choices.

- Uses advanced knowledge of pharmacology, psychoneuroimmunology, nutritional supplements, herbal and homeopathic remedies, and a variety of complementary and alternative therapies in prescribing.

- Evaluates and incorporates complementary/alternative/integrative therapies into education and practice.

- Prescribes holistic therapies that enhance body-mind-emotion-spirit-environment connectedness and foster healing and wholeness.

- Evaluates therapeutic and potential adverse effects of pharmacological and nonpharmacological treatments, including but not limited to drug/herbal/homeopathic regimens, as well as drug/herbal/homeopathic side effects and interactions.

- Provides individuals with information about intended effects and potential adverse effects of proposed prescriptive therapies.

- Provides information about costs and alternative treatments and procedures, as appropriate.

Standard 6. Evaluation

The holistic registered nurse evaluates progress toward attainment of outcomes while recognizing and honoring the continuing holistic nature of the healing process.

COMPETENCIES

The holistic registered nurse:

- Conducts a holistic, systematic, ongoing, and criterion-based evaluation of the outcomes in relation to the structures and processes prescribed by the plan and the indicated timeline.

- Analyzes the effects of single and multiple interventions on the person's health and functioning.

- Collaborates with the person and others involved in the care or situation in the evaluative process.

- Assesses the person's, family's, and significant other's understanding of the diagnosis, issue, plan, and options.

- Evaluates, in partnership with the person, the effectiveness of the planned strategies in relation to the person's responses and the attainment of the expected and unfolding outcomes.

- Uses ongoing assessment data to mutually revise, with the person, family, and health team, the diagnoses, outcomes, plan, and implementation, as needed.

- Disseminates the results to the person, family, and others involved in accordance with state and federal laws and regulations.

- Participates in assessing and assuring the responsible and appropriate use of interventions in order to minimize unwarranted or unwanted treatment and healthcare consumer suffering.

- Documents the results of the evaluation.

ADDITIONAL COMPETENCIES FOR THE GRADUATE-LEVEL-PREPARED HOLISTIC NURSE AND THE APRN

The graduate-level-prepared holistic nurse or the advanced practice registered nurse:

- Evaluates, in partnership with the person, the accuracy of the diagnosis and the effectiveness of the interventions in relationship to the person's attainment of expected and evolving outcomes and changes of meaning in the person's health experience.

- Synthesizes the results of the evaluation to determine the effect of the plan on the affected individuals, families, groups, communities, and institutions.

- Adapts the plan of care for the trajectory of treatment according to evaluation of response.

- Uses the results of the evaluation analyses to make or recommend process or structural changes, including policy, procedure, and/or protocol revision, as appropriate to improve holistic care.

Standards of Professional Performance

Standard 7. Ethics

The holistic registered nurse practices ethically.

COMPETENCIES

The holistic registered nurse:

- Uses *Code of Ethics for Nurses with Interpretative Statements* (ANA, 2001) and *Position Statement on Holistic Nursing Ethics* (AHNA, 2007) to guide practice and articulate the moral foundation of holistic nursing.

- Identifies the ethic of caring and its contribution to unity of self, others, nature, and God/Life Force/Absolute/Transcendent as central to holistic nursing practice.

- Delivers care in a manner that preserves and protects the person's uniqueness, autonomy, dignity, rights, values, and beliefs.

- Recognizes the centrality of the person and family as core members of any healthcare team.

- Upholds the person's personal privacy and confidentiality within legal and regulatory parameters.

- Assists the person in developing skills for self-advocacy, self-determination, and informed decision-making about his/her care.

- Respects the person's choices and health trajectory, which may be incongruent with conventional wisdom.

- Maintains a therapeutic and professional person–nurse relationship within appropriate professional role boundaries.

- Contributes to resolving ethical issues involving healthcare consumers, colleagues, community groups, systems, and/or other stakeholders.

- Takes appropriate action regarding instances of illegal, unethical, or inappropriate behavior that could endanger or jeopardize the best interests of the healthcare consumer or situation.

- Speaks up when appropriate to question healthcare practice, when necessary for safety and quality improvement.

- Advocates for equitable consumer healthcare, particularly regarding the rights of vulnerable, repressed, or underserved populations, by such activities as:

  - Acting on behalf of individuals, families, groups, and communities who cannot seek or demand ethical treatment on their own

  - Seeking to eliminate barriers such as affordability and accessibility that create added risks for persons of varied racial, ethnic, social backgrounds, as well as older adults and children

  - Advocating for other nurses and colleagues

- Recognizes that the well-being of the ecosystem of the planet is a determining condition for the well-being of humans.

- Demonstrates a commitment to self-reflection and self-assessment and to practicing self-care strategies to enhance physical, psychological, intellectual, sociological, and spiritual well-being, manage stress, and connect with self and others.

- Values all life experiences as opportunities to find personal meaning and cultivate self-awareness, self-reflection, and growth.

ADDITIONAL COMPETENCIES FOR THE GRADUATE-LEVEL-PREPARED HOLISTIC NURSE AND THE APRN

The graduate-level-prepared holistic nurse or the advanced practice registered nurse:

- Participates in interprofessional teams that address ethical risks, benefits, and outcomes.

- Provides information on the risks, benefits, and outcomes of healthcare regimens to allow informed decision-making by the healthcare consumer, including informed consent and informed refusal.

- Engages others to incorporate a holistic perspective of ethical situations and decision-making.

- Actively contributes to creating an ecosystem that supports well-being for all life.

Standard 8. Education

The holistic registered nurse attains knowledge and competence that reflect current nursing practice.

COMPETENCIES

The holistic registered nurse:

- Participates in ongoing educational activities related to appropriate knowledge bases for holistic care and professional issues.

- Demonstrates a commitment to lifelong learning through self-reflection and inquiry to identify learning and personal growth needs.

- Seeks experiences that reflect current practice in order to maintain knowledge, skills, abilities, and judgment in clinical practice or holistic role performance.

- Acquires knowledge and skills appropriate to the holistic nursing specialty, role, population, practice setting, or situation.

- Identifies learning needs based on nursing knowledge, the various roles the holistic nurse may assume, the changing needs of the population, and personal growth.

- Educates others by demonstrating a holistic philosophy and ethic that value all ways of knowing and learning.

- Seeks experiences and formal and independent learning activities to develop and maintain clinical and professional skills and knowledge and personal growth.

- Participates in formal or informal consultations to address issues in holistic nursing practice as an application of education and knowledge base.

- Shares educational findings, knowledge, experiences, and ideas with peers.

- Contributes to a work environment conducive to the education of healthcare professionals.

- Maintains professional records that provide evidence of competence and lifelong learning.

ADDITIONAL COMPETENCIES FOR THE GRADUATE-LEVEL-PREPARED HOLISTIC NURSE AND THE APRN

The graduate-level-prepared holistic nurse or the advanced practice registered nurse:

- Uses current healthcare research findings and other evidence to expand clinical knowledge, skills, abilities, and judgment; to enhance holistic role performance; and to increase knowledge of professional issues and changes in national standards for practice and trends in holistic care.

Standard 9. Evidence-Based Practice and Research

The holistic registered nurse integrates evidence and research findings into practice.

COMPETENCIES

The holistic registered nurse:

- Utilizes the best available evidence, including current evidence-based nursing knowledge, theories, and research findings, to guide practice.

- Incorporates evidence when initiating changes in nursing practice.

- Actively and ethically participates, as appropriate to education level and position, in the formulation of evidence-based practice through research related to holistic health. Such activities may include:

  - Identifying problems specific to nursing research (person care and nursing practice)

  - Participating in data collection

  - Participating in a formal committee or program

  - Sharing research activities and/or findings with individuals/families/peers, those in other disciplines, and others

  - Systematically inquiring into healing, wholeness, cultural, spiritual, and health issues by conducting research or supporting and utilizing the research of others

  - Critically analyzing and interpreting research for application to holistic practice

  - Using research findings in the development of policies, procedures, and standards of practice in holistic person care

  - Incorporating research as a basis for learning

- Shares personal or third-party research findings with colleagues and peers.

ADDITIONAL COMPETENCIES FOR THE GRADUATE-LEVEL-PREPARED HOLISTIC NURSE AND THE APRN

The graduate-level-prepared holistic nurse or the advanced practice registered nurse:

- Contributes to nursing knowledge by conducting or synthesizing research that discovers, examines, and evaluates current practice, knowledge, theories, philosophies, context, criteria, and creative approaches to improve holistic healthcare outcomes.

- Promotes a climate of research and clinical inquiry.

- Disseminates research findings through activities such as presentations, publications, consultations, and journal clubs for a variety of audiences (including nursing, other disciplines, and the public) to improve holistic care and further develop the foundation and practice of holistic nursing.

- Creates ways to study the integration of body-mind-emotion-spirit-environment therapies to achieve optimal care outcomes.

- Participates with others to identify research questions or areas for inquiry and set research priorities that have high significance in understanding and/or improving health/wellness promotion and disease prevention; the quality of life; spirituality; cultural beliefs and health practices; healing and well-being; and whole-health and whole systems of care.

Standard 10. Quality of Practice

The holistic registered nurse contributes to quality nursing practice.

COMPETENCIES

The holistic registered nurse:

- Demonstrates quality by documenting the application of the nursing process in a responsible, accountable, and ethical manner.

- Uses creativity and innovation to enhance holistic nursing care.

- Obtains and maintains professional certification if it is available in the area of expertise.

- Participates in quality improvement activities for holistic nursing practice. Activities may include:

  - Identifying aspects of practice important for quality monitoring

  - Using indicators developed to monitor quality and effectiveness of holistic nursing practice

  - Collecting data to monitor quality and effectiveness of holistic nursing practice

  - Analyzing quality data to identify opportunities for improving holistic nursing practice

  - Formulating recommendations to improve holistic nursing practice or outcomes

  - Implementing activities to enhance the quality of holistic nursing practice

  - Developing, implementing, and/or evaluating policies, procedures, and/or guidelines to improve the quality of practice

  - Participating on and/or leading interprofessional teams to evaluate clinical care or health services

  - Participating in and/or leading efforts to minimize costs and unnecessary duplication

- Identifying problems that occur in day-to-day work routines so that process inefficiencies may be corrected

- Analyzing factors related to quality, safety, satisfaction, and effectiveness

- Analyzing organizational systems for barriers to quality healthcare consumer outcomes

- Implementing processes to remove or decrease barriers to holistic care within organizational systems

- Working toward creating organizations that value sacred space and environments that enhance healing

ADDITIONAL COMPETENCIES FOR THE GRADUATE-LEVEL-PREPARED HOLISTIC NURSE AND THE APRN

The graduate-level-prepared holistic nurse or the advanced practice registered nurse:

- Provides leadership in the design and implementation of quality improvements for holistic care.

- Designs innovations to effect change in practice and improve holistic health outcomes.

- Evaluates the practice environment and quality of holistic nursing care rendered in relation to existing evidence and feedback from individuals, families, and significant others.

- Identifies opportunities for the generation and use of research and evidence.

- Obtains and maintains professional certification if it is available in the area of expertise.

- Uses the results of quality improvement to initiate changes in holistic nursing practice and the healthcare delivery system.

Standard 11. Communication

The holistic registered nurse communicates effectively in a variety of formats in all areas of practice.

COMPETENCIES

The holistic registered nurse:

- Assesses communication format preferences of individuals, families, significant others, and colleagues.

- Assesses her/his own communication skills and effects in encounters with individuals, families, significant others, and colleagues.

- Uses intention, centering, presence, caring, intuition, and deep listening in creating and maintaining healing and person-centered communication.

- Seeks continuous improvement of her/his own communication and conflict-management/resolution skills.

- Conveys information to individuals, families, significant others, the interprofessional team, and others in communication formats that promote accuracy, respect, authenticity, and trust.

- Questions the rationale supporting care processes and decisions when they do not appear to be in the best interest of the person.

- Discloses observations or concerns related to hazards and errors in care or the practice environment to the appropriate level.

- Maintains communication with other providers to minimize risks associated with transfers and transition in care delivery.

- Contributes her/his own professional perspective in discussions with the interprofessional team.

- Promotes work environments conducive to support, understanding, respect, health, healing, caring, wholeness, and harmony.

ADDITIONAL COMPETENCIES FOR THE GRADUATE-LEVEL-PREPARED HOLISTIC NURSE AND THE APRN

The graduate-level-prepared holistic nurse or the advanced practice registered nurse:

- Establishes practice environments that recognize and value holistic communication as fundamental to holistic care.

Standard 12. Leadership

The holistic registered nurse demonstrates leadership in the professional practice setting and the profession.

COMPETENCIES

The holistic registered nurse:

- Oversees the nursing care given by others while retaining accountability for the quality of care given to the healthcare consumer.

- Abides by the vision, the associated goals, and the plan to implement and measure the holistic healthcare progress of the person or progress within the context of the healthcare organization.

- Demonstrates a commitment to continuous, lifelong learning, education, and personal growth for self and others.

- Mentors colleagues for the advancement of holistic nursing practice, the profession, and quality holistic health care.

- Communicates effectively with individuals, families, significant others, and colleagues.

- Treats colleagues with respect, trust, and dignity.

- Develops communication and conflict-management/resolution skills.

- Exhibits transformational leadership by:

  - Dealing with ambiguity and exhibiting creativity and flexibility through times of change

  - Demonstrating energy, excitement, and a passion for quality holistic work

  - Seeking ways to advance nursing autonomy and accountability

  - Creating a culture in which risk-taking is both safe and expected

  - Valuing people as the most precious asset in an organization

- Promotes advancement of the profession through participation in professional organizations and focus on strategies that bring unity and healing to the nursing profession.

■ Participates in efforts to influence healthcare policy involving healthcare consumers and the profession.

■ Seeks to advance nursing autonomy and accountability and the philosophy and practice of holistic care by participating on committees, councils, and administrative teams.

■ Engages at local, state, national, and international levels to expand the knowledge and practice of holistic nursing and awareness of holistic health issues.

ADDITIONAL COMPETENCIES FOR THE GRADUATE-LEVEL-PREPARED HOLISTIC NURSE AND THE APRN

The graduate-level-prepared holistic nurse or the advanced practice registered nurse:

■ Influences decision-making bodies to improve holistic integrative care, the professional practice environment, and holistic healthcare consumer outcomes.

■ Provides direction to enhance the effectiveness of the interprofessional team.

■ Promotes advanced practice in holistic nursing and role development by interpreting the role to healthcare consumers, families, and others.

■ Models expert holistic practice to interprofessional team members and healthcare consumers.

■ Mentors colleagues in the acquisition of holistic clinical knowledge, skills, abilities, and judgment.

■ Articulates the ideas underpinning holistic nursing philosophy, placing these ideas in a historical, philosophical, and scientific context while projecting future trends in thinking by such activities as:

■ Applying, teaching, mentoring, and leading others in developing holistic care models

■ Leading organizations in creating therapeutic healing environments that value holistic caring, social support, and healing, where individuals feel connected, supported, and valued

- Promoting communication of information and advancement of the profession and holistic nursing through writing, publishing, and presentations for professional or lay/public audiences

- Understanding the political, social, organizational, and financial barriers to holistic care for individuals, population groups, and communities and working to eliminate these barriers while balancing justice with compassion

- Sharing knowledge and understanding of a wide range of cultural norms and healthcare practices/beliefs/values concerning individuals, families, groups, and communities from varied racial, ethnic, spiritual, and social backgrounds

Standard 13. Collaboration

The holistic registered nurse collaborates with the healthcare consumer, family, and others in the conduct of holistic nursing practice.

COMPETENCIES

The holistic registered nurse:

- Recognizes expertise and competence of diverse disciplines and approaches to health care.

- Partners with others to effect change, enhance holistic care, and produce positive outcomes through the sharing of knowledge of the person and/or the situation.

- Communicates with the person, family, significant others, caregivers, and interdisciplinary healthcare providers regarding the person's care and the holistic nurse's role in the provision of that care.

- Engages in teamwork and team-building processes.

- Promotes engagement by participating in consensus building and /or resolving conflict in the context of person-/relationship-centered care.

- Applies group process and negotiation techniques with healthcare consumers and colleagues.

- Adheres to standards and applicable codes of conduct governing behavior among peers and colleagues to create a work environment that promotes cooperation, respect, and trust.

- Cooperates in creating a documented plan that is focused on holistic outcomes and decisions related to care and delivery of services, which indicates communication with individuals receiving care, families, and others.

- Incorporates a range of approaches and therapies from diverse disciplines and systems of care as appropriate.

ADDITIONAL COMPETENCIES FOR THE GRADUATE-LEVEL-PREPARED HOLISTIC NURSE AND THE APRN

The graduate-level-prepared holistic nurse or the advanced practice registered nurse:

- Partners with other disciplines to enhance holistic care and outcomes through interprofessional activities such as education, consultation, referral management, technological development, or research opportunities.

- Facilitates the contribution of the healthcare consumer, family, significant others, and team members in order to achieve optimal outcomes.

- Leads in establishing, improving, and sustaining collaborative relationships to achieve safe, quality, holistic, person-centered care.

- Documents plan-of-care communications, rationales for plan-of-care changes, and collaborative discussions to improve holistic healthcare outcomes.

- Facilitates the negotiation of holistic/complementary/alternative/integrative and conventional healthcare services for continuity of care and program planning.

Standard 14. Professional Practice Evaluation

The holistic registered nurse evaluates her/his own nursing practice in relation to professional practice standards and guidelines, relevant statutes, rules, and regulations.

COMPETENCIES

The holistic registered nurse:

- Reflects on his/her practice and how his/her own personal, cultural, and/or spiritual beliefs, experiences, biases, education, and values may affect care given to individuals, families, and communities.

- Provides age and developmentally appropriate care in a culturally and ethnically sensitive manner.

- Engages in self-evaluation of practice on a regular basis, identifying areas of strength as well as areas in which professional development and personal growth would be beneficial.

- Obtains informal feedback regarding her/his own holistic practice from individuals receiving care, peers, professional colleagues, and others.

- Participates in peer review as appropriate.

- Takes action to achieve goals identified through the evaluation process.

- Provides the evidence for practice beliefs, decisions, and actions as part of the informal and formal evaluation processes.

- Interacts with peers and colleagues to enhance her/his own professional nursing practice or holistic role performance.

- Provides peers with formal or informal constructive feedback regarding their practice or role performance.

ADDITIONAL COMPETENCIES FOR THE GRADUATE-LEVEL-PREPARED HOLISTIC NURSE AND THE APRN

The graduate-level-prepared holistic nurse or the advanced practice registered nurse:

- Engages in a formal process of seeking feedback regarding his/her own practice from individuals receiving care, peers, professional colleagues, and others.

Standard 15. Resource Utilization

The holistic registered nurse utilizes appropriate resources to plan and provide nursing services that are holistic, safe, effective, and financially responsible.

COMPETENCIES

The holistic registered nurse:

- Assesses the person's and family's care needs and resources available to achieve desired outcomes.

- Identifies the person's care needs, potential for harm, complexity of the task, and desired outcomes when considering resource allocation.

- Delegates elements of care to appropriate healthcare workers in accordance with any applicable legal or policy parameters or principles.

- Identifies the evidence when evaluating resources.

- Advocates for resources, including technology, that enhance holistic nursing practice.

- Modifies practice when necessary to promote positive interaction between the person, care providers, and technology.

- Assists the person, family, significant others, and caregivers, as appropriate, in identifying and securing appropriate and available services to address needs across the healthcare continuum.

- Assists the person, family, and significant others in becoming informed consumers about health options and factoring costs, risks, and benefits in decisions about treatment and care.

- Identifies discriminatory healthcare practices and their impact.

- Engages in effective nondiscriminatory practices.

ADDITIONAL COMPETENCIES FOR THE GRADUATE-LEVEL-PREPARED HOLISTIC NURSE AND THE APRN

The graduate-level-prepared holistic nurse or the advanced practice registered nurse:

- Utilizes organizational and community resources to formulate interprofessional plans of care.

- Formulates innovative solutions for healthcare consumer care problems that utilize resources effectively and maintain quality.

- Designs evaluation strategies that demonstrate cost effectiveness, cost benefit, and efficiency factors associated with holistic nursing practice.

Standard 16. Environmental Health

The holistic registered nurse practices in an environmentally safe and healthy manner.

COMPETENCIES

The holistic registered nurse:

- Attains knowledge of environmental health concepts, such as implementation of environmental health strategies.

- Promotes a practice environment that reduces environmental health risks for workers and healthcare consumers.

- Assesses the practice environment for factors that threaten health, such as sound, odor, noise, and light.

- Advocates for the judicious and appropriate use of products in health care.

- Communicates environmental health risks and exposure reduction strategies to healthcare consumers, families, colleagues, and communities.

- Utilizes scientific evidence to determine if a product or treatment is an environmental threat.

- Participates in strategies to promote healthy communities.

- Engages in activities that respect, nurture, and enhance the integral relationship with the earth, and advocates for the well-being of the global community's economy, education, and social justice.

ADDITIONAL COMPETENCIES FOR THE GRADUATE-LEVEL-PREPARED HOLISTIC NURSE AND THE APRN

The graduate-level-prepared holistic nurse or the advanced practice registered nurse:

- Creates partnerships that promote sustainable environmental health policies and conditions.

- Analyzes the impact of social, political, and economic influences on the environment and human health exposures.

- Contributes to conducting research and applying research findings that link environmental hazards and human response patterns.

- Critically evaluates the manner in which environmental health issues are presented by the popular media.

- Advocates for implementation of environmental principles for nursing practice.

- Supports nurses in advocating for and implementing environmental principles in nursing practice.

- Acts as a leader, collaborator, consultant, and change agent in evaluating global health issues and environmental safety; anticipating the potential effect of environmental hazards on the health or welfare of individuals, groups, and communities; and assisting in reducing or eliminating environmental hazards.

Glossary

Allopathic/conventional therapies. Medical, surgical, pharmacological, and invasive and noninvasive diagnostic procedures; those interventions most commonly used in allopathic, Western medicine.

Complementary/alternative/integrative modalities (CAM). A broad set of healthcare practices, therapies, and modalities that address the whole person—body, mind, emotion, spirit—rather than just signs and symptoms, which can replace or may be used as complements to conventional Western medical, surgical, and pharmacological treatments.

Critical thinking. An active, purposeful, organized cognitive process involving creativity, reflection, problem-solving, both rational and intuitive judgment, an attitude of inquiry, and a philosophical orientation toward thinking about thinking.

Cultural competence. The ability to deliver health care with knowledge of and sensitivity to cultural factors that influence the health behavior, curing, healing, dying, and the grieving process of the person.

Environment. The context of habitat within which all living systems participate and interact, including the physical body and its physical habitat along with the cultural, psychological, social, and historical influences; includes both the external physical space and the person's internal physical, mental, emotional, social, and spiritual experience.

Evidence-based practice. The process by which integrative healthcare practitioners make clinical decisions using the best integrative philosophy and theories, research evidence, clinical expertise, and patient preferences within the context of available resources.

Healing. A lifelong journey into wholeness, seeking harmony, balance, and right relationship in one's own life and in family, community, and global relations. Healing involves those physical, mental, social, and spiritual processes of recovery, repair, renewal, and transformation that increase wholeness and often (though not invariably) order and coherence. Healing is an emergent process of the whole system bringing together aspects of one's self and the body-mind-emotion-spirit-environment at deeper levels of inner knowing, leading toward integration and balance, with each aspect having equal importance and value. Healing can lead to more complex levels of personal understanding and meaning, and may be synchronous but not synonymous with curing.

Healing process. A continual journey of change and evolution of one's self through life, characterized by the awareness of patterns that support or are challenges/barriers to health and healing; may be undertaken alone or in a healing community.

Healing relationships. The quality and characteristics of interactions between one who facilitates healing and the person who is in the process of healing. Characteristics of such interactions involve empathy, caring, love, warmth, trust, confidence, credibility, competence, honesty, courtesy, respect, sharing of expectations, and good communication.

Healing system. A true healthcare system in which people can receive adequate, nontoxic, and noninvasive assistance in maintaining wellness and healing for body, mind, emotion, and spirit, together with the most sophisticated, aggressive, curing technologies available.

Health. An individually defined state or process in which the individual (nurse, client, family, group, or community) experiences a sense of well-being, harmony, and unity such that subjective experiences about health, health beliefs, and values are honored; a process of becoming and expanding consciousness.

Health promotion. Activities and preventive measures to promote health, increase well-being, and actualize human potential of people, families, communities, society, and ecology; examples include immunizations, fitness/exercise programs, breast self-exam, appropriate nutrition, relaxation, stress management, social support, prayer, meditation, healing rituals, cultural practices, and promoting environmental health and safety.

Holistic communication. A caring–healing process that calls forth the full use of self in interacting with another. A free flow of verbal and nonverbal interchange between and among people and significant beings such as pets, nature, and God/Life Force/Absolute/Transcendent that explores meaning and ideas leading to mutual understanding and growth.

Holistic ethics. The basic underlying concept of the unity and integral wholeness of all people and of all nature, identified and pursued by finding unity and wholeness within the self and within humanity. In this framework, acts are not performed for the sake of law, precedent, or social norms, but rather from a desire to do good freely in order to witness, identify, and contribute to unity.

Holistic healing. A form of healing based on attention to all aspects of an individual: physical, mental, emotional, sexual, cultural, social, spiritual, and energetic; the manifestation of the right relationship at one or more levels of the body-mind-emotion-spirit-energy system.

Holistic nurse. A nurse who recognizes and integrates body-mind-emotion-spirit-energy-environment principles and modalities in daily life and clinical practice, creates a caring healing space within herself/himself that allows the nurse to be an instrument of healing, shares authenticity of unconditional presence that helps to remove the barriers to the healing process, facilitates another person's growth (body-mind-emotion-spirit-energy-environment connections), and assists with recovery from illness or transition to peaceful death.

Holistic nursing practice process. An iterative and integrative process involving six steps that may occur simultaneously: (1) assessing, (2) diagnosing or identifying patterns/challenges/needs/health issue(s), (3) identifying outcomes, (4) planning care, (5) implementing the plan of care, and (6) evaluating.

Honor. An act or intention indicating the holding of self or another in high respect, esteem, and dignity, including valuing and accepting the humanity of people, with regard for the decisions and wishes of another.

Human caring. The moral ideal of nursing, in which the nurse brings her/his whole self into a relationship with the whole self of the person being cared for in order to protect that person's vulnerability, preserve the person's humanity and dignity, and reinforce the meaning and experience of oneness and unity.

Human health experience. The totality of human experience, including each person's subjective experience about health, health beliefs, illness, values, sexual orientation, and personal preferences, that encompasses health-wellness-disease-illness-death.

Illness. A subjective experience of symptoms and suffering to which the individual ascribes meaning and significance; not synonymous with disease; a shift in the homeodynamic balance of the person to disharmony and imbalance.

Intention. The conscious awareness of being in the present moment to help facilitate the healing process; a volitional act of love.

Interdisciplinary/interprofessional. Conversation or collaboration across disciplines in which knowledge is shared that informs learning, practice, education, and research; includes individuals, families, community members, and other disciplines.

Meaning. That which is signified, indicated, referred to, or understood. More specifically: *Philosophical meaning*: Meaning that depends on the symbolic connections that are grasped by reason. *Psychological meaning*: Meaning that depends on connections experienced through intuition or insight.

Person. An individual, client, healthcare consumer, patient, family member, significant other, support person, or community member who has the opportunity to engage in interaction with a holistic nurse.

Person-centered care. The human caring process in which the holistic nurse gives full attention and intention to the whole self of a person, not merely the current presenting symptoms, illness, crisis, or tasks to be accomplished, and that includes reinforcing the person's meaning and experience of oneness and unity; the created condition of trust in which holistic care can be given and received.

Presence. The essential state or core of healing; approaching an individual in a way that respects and honors her/his essence; relating in a way that reflects a quality of being with and in collaboration/partnership with rather than doing to; entering into a shared experience (or field of consciousness) that promotes healing potential and an experience of well-being.

Relationship-centered care. A process model of caregiving that is based in a vision of community where three types of relationships are identified: (1) patient–practitioner relationship, (2) community–practitioner relationship, and (3) practitioner–practitioner relationship. Each of these interrelated relationships is essential within a reformed integrative healthcare delivery system in a hospital, clinic, community, or home. Each component involves a unique set of responsibilities and tasks that addresses three areas: knowledge, values, and skills (Tresolini & Pew-Fetzer Task Force, 1994).

Spirituality. The feelings, thoughts, experiences, and behaviors that arise from a search for meaning. That which is generally considered sacred or holy. Usually, though not universally, considered to involve a sense of connection with an absolute, imminent, or transcendent spiritual force, however named, as well as the conviction that meaning, value, direction, and purpose are valid aspects of the individual and universe. The essence of being and relatedness that permeates all of life and is manifested in one's knowing, doing, and being. The interconnectedness with self, others, nature, and God/Life Force/Absolute/Transcendent. Not necessarily synonymous with religion.

Transformational leadership. Leadership that creates valuable and positive change in individuals and systems, encouraging individuals to contribute to their fullest potential by enhancing the motivation, morale, and performance of followers.

Transpersonal. A personal understanding that is based on one's experiences of temporarily transcending or moving beyond one's usual identification with the limited biological, historical, cultural, and personal self at the deepest and most profound levels of experience possible. From this perspective, the ordinary, biological, historical, cultural, and personal self is seen as an important but only a partial manifestation or expression of this much greater something that is one's deeper origin and destination. That which transcends the limits and boundaries of individual ego identities and possibilities to include acknowledgment and appreciation of something greater.

Wellness. Integrated, congruent functioning aimed toward reaching one's highest potential.

Many of the definitions in this document were adapted from *Holistic Nursing: Scope and Standards of Practice* (AHNA & ANA, 2007), and Dossey and Keegan (2013), with permission.

References and Bibliography

AARP/NCCAM. (2011). *Complementary and alternative medicine: What people aged 50 and older discuss with their health care providers.* Washington, DC: U.S. DHHS.

Administration on Aging, Department of Health and Human Services. (2011). *Aging statistics.* Available at www.aoa.gov/aging statistics

American Association of Colleges of Nursing (AACN). (2008). *The essentials of baccalaureate education for professional nursing practice.* Washington, DC: AACN.

American Association of Colleges of Nursing. (2011). Nursing shortage (AACN Fact Sheet, April, 2011). Available from http://www.aacn.nche.edu/media/factsheets

American Holistic Nurses Association. (1998). *Description of holistic nursing.* Flagstaff, AZ: AHNA.

American Holistic Nurses Association. (2009). *White paper: Research in AHNA.* Flagstaff, AZ: AHNA.

American Holistic Nurses Association. (2012). *Position statement on holistic nursing ethics.* Flagstaff, AZ: AHNA.

American Holistic Nurses Association & American Nurses Association. (2007). *Holistic nursing: Scope and standards of practice.* Silver Spring, MD: Nursesbooks.org.

American Nurses Association. (2001). *Code of Ethics for Nurses with interpretive statements.* Silver Spring, MD: Nursesbooks.org.

American Nurses Association. (2004). *Nursing: Scope and standards of practice.* Silver Spring, MD: Nursesbooks.org.

American Nurses Association. (2010a). *Guide to the Code of Ethics for Nurses: Interpretation and application.* Silver Spring, MD: Nursesbooks.org.

American Nurses Association. (2010b). *Nursing: Scope and standards of practice*, 2nd ed. Silver Spring, MD: Nursesbooks.org.

American Nurses Association. (2010c). *Nursing's social policy statement: The essence of the profession.* Silver Spring, MD: Nursesbooks.org.

APRN Consensus Work Group & National Council of State Boards of Nursing APRN Advisory Committee. (2008). *Consensus model for APRN regulation: Licensure, accreditation, certification and education.* Available at http://www.nursingworld.org/ConsensusModelforAPRN

Barnes, P. M., Bloom, B., & Nahin, B. R. (2008). Complementary and alternative medicine use among adults and children: United States, 2007. *CDC National Health Statistics Reports, 12.*

Benner, P., Sutphen, M., Leonard, V., & Day, L. (2010). *Educating nurses: A call for radical transformation.* San Francisco, CA: Jossey-Bass.

Bezold, C. (2011, April 25). Alert: Major study on future of primary care seeks input on IM therapies and CAM practitioners. *Integrator Blog.* Available at http://theintegratorblog.com/index.php?option=com_content&task=view&id=744&Itemid=189

Buerhaus, P., Auerbach, D., & Staiger, D. (2009). The recent surge in nurse employment: Causes and implications. *Health Affairs, 28*(4), 657–668.

Centers for Disease Control and Prevention. (2011, May 11). *Chronic disease prevention and health promotion.* Available at http://www.cdc.gov/chronicdisease/index.htm

Cowling, W. R. (2011). Holism as a sociopolitical enterprise. *Journal of Holistic Nursing, 29*(1), 5–6.

Dossey, B. (2010). Holistic nursing: From Florence Nightingale's historical legacy to 21st-century global nursing. *Alternative Therapies in Health & Medicine, 16*(5), 14–16.

Dossey, B., & Keegan, L. (Eds.). (2013). *Holistic nursing: A handbook for practice*, 6th ed. Sudbury, MA: Jones & Bartlett.

Eisenberg, D. M., Kessler, R. C., Foster, C., Norlock, F. E., Calkins, D. R., & Delbanco, T. L. (1993). Unconventional medicine in the United States: Prevalence, costs, and patterns of use. *New England Journal of Medicine, 328*(4), 246–252. (Abstract and citations available at http://content.nejm .org/cgi/content/abstract/328/4/246)

Eisenberg, D., Davis, R. B., Ettner, S. L., Appel, S., Wiilke, S., Van Rompay, M., & Kessler, R. C. (1998). Trends in alternative medicine use in the United States, 1990–1997. *Journal of the American Medical Association, 280*, 1569–1575.

Eliopolous, C. (2009). *Nurse competency in aging: Safe integration of complementary and alternative therapies in geriatric care.* Flagstaff, AZ: AHNA.

Fenton, M., & Morris, D. (2003). The integration of holistic nursing practices and complementary and alternative modalities into curricula of schools of nursing. *Alternative Therapies in Health & Nursing, 9*(4), 62–67.

Goldblatt, E., Snider, P., Quinn, S., & Weeks, J. (2009). *Clinicians' and educators' desk reference on the licensed complementary and alternative healthcare professions.* Seattle, WA: ACCAHC.

HealthCare Problems.org. (2011, September). *Health care statistics.* Available at http://www.healthcareproblems.org

Health Forum & Samueli Institute. (2010). *Complementary and alternative medicine survey of hospitals summary of results.* Alexandria, VA: Samueli Institute.

Hyman, M. (2005). Quality in health care: Asking the right questions. The next ten years: The role of CAM in the "quality cure." *Alternative Therapies in Health & Medicine, 11*(3), 18–19.

Institute of Medicine. (2005). *Complementary and alternative medicine in the United States.* Washington, DC: National Academies Press.

Institute of Medicine. (2009). *Summit on integrative medicine and the health of the public.* Washington, DC: National Academy of Sciences.

Institute of Medicine. (2010). *The future of nursing: Leading change, advancing health*. Washington, DC: National Academies Press. Available at http://www.iom.edu/nursing

KaiserEdu.org. (2010, March). *U.S. health care costs: Background brief.* Available at http://www.kaiseredu.org/Issue-Modules /US-Health-Care-Costs

Lee, R. (2010). The new pandemic: Superstress? *Explore: The Journal of Science & Healing, 6*(1), 7–10.

Levin, J., & Reich, J. (2013). Self-reflection. In B. Dossey and L. Keegan (Eds.), *Holistic nursing: A handbook for practice*, 6th ed. (pp. 247–260). Sudbury, MA: Jones & Bartlett.

Luck, S., & Keegan, L. (2013). Environmental health. In B. Dossey and L. Keegan (Eds.), *Holistic nursing: A handbook for practice*, 6th ed. (pp. 633–671). Sudbury, MA: Jones & Bartlett.

Mariano, C. (2007). The nursing shortage: Is stress management the answer? *Beginnings, 27*(1), 3.

Mariano, C. (2008). Contributions to holism through critique of theory and research. *Beginnings, 28*(2), 26.

Mariano, C. (2013). Current trends and issues in holistic nursing. In B. Dossey and L. Keegan (Eds.), *Holistic nursing: A handbook for practice*, 6th ed. (pp. 85–106). Sudbury, MA: Jones & Bartlett.

Mittleman, M., Alperson, S. Y., Arcari, P., Donnelly, G., Ford, L., Koithan, M., & Kreitzer, M. J. (2010). Nursing and integrative health care. *Alternative Therapies in Health & Medicine, 16*(5), 74–84.

National Center for Complementary and Alternative Medicine (NCCAM). (2009, July 30). Americans spent $33.9 billion out-of-pocket on complementary and alternative medicine. Available at http://nccam.nih .gov/news/2009/073009.htm

National Center for Complementary and Alternative Medicine (NCCAM). (2011a). *Categories of complementary/alternative modalities (CAM) therapies*. Available at http://nccam.nih.gov

National Center for Complementary and Alternative Medicine (NCCAM). (2011b). *Exploring the science of complementary and alternative medicine: Third strategic plan 2011–2015.* Washington, DC: U.S. Department of Health and Human Services, National Institutes of Health.

Nursing Interventions Classification (NIC). (n.d.). *NIC labels and definitions.* Available at http://www.nursing.uiowa.edu/sites/default/files/documents /cncce/LabelDefinitionsNIC5.pdf or http://www.nursing.uiowa.edu /cncce/nic-labels-and-definitions [based on Bulechek, G. M., Butcher, H. K., & Dochterman, J. C. (Eds.). (2008). *Nursing Interventions Classification (NIC)*, 5th ed. St. Louis, MO: Mosby Elsevier].

Public Agenda. (2011, May 11). Half of Americans say the health care system has major problems. Available at http://www.publicagenda.org/charts /half-americans-say-health-care-system-has-major-problems-and-most -say-it-needs-be-fundamentally-changed-or

Quinn, J. (2013). Transpersonal human caring and healing. In B. Dossey and L. Keegan (Eds.), *Holistic nursing: A handbook for practice*, 6th ed. (pp. 107–116). Sudbury, MA: Jones & Bartlett.

Robert Wood Johnson Foundation. (2012). *RN work project.* Available at www.rnworkproject.org

Samueli Institute. (2009). *A wellness initiative for the nation (WIN).* Available at http://www.lifesciencefoundation.org/WellnessInitiative11feb09.pdf

Tresolini, C. P., & Pew-Fetzer Task Force. (1994). *Health professions education and relationship-centered care: Report of the Pew-Fetzer Task Force on advancing psychosocial education.* San Francisco, CA: Pew Health Professions Commission. Available at http://www.futurehealth.ucsf.edu /pdf_files/RelationshipCentered.pdf

Tu, H., Boukus, E., & Cohen, G. (2010/2012). Workplace clinics: A sign of growing employer interest in wellness. *Health Systems Change* (HSC Research Brief 17). Washington, DC: Center for Studying Health System Change.

U.S. Census Bureau. (2011). *Statistical abstract of the United States: 2011.* Washington, DC: Author.

U.S. Centers for Medicare and Medicaid Services, Office of the Actuary. Available at http://www.cms.hhs.gov/NationalHealthExpendData

U.S. Department of Health and Human Services. (1999). *The patient's bill of rights in Medicare and Medicaid*. Available at http://www.hhs.gov/news /press/1999pres/990412.html

U.S. Department of Health and Human Services. (2010). *Healthy people 2020*. Washington, DC: Author. Available at http://www.healthypeople.gov

U.S. Office of the Surgeon General. (2011). *The national prevention and health promotion strategy (National Prevention Strategy)*. Washington, DC: U.S. Department of Health and Human Services.

Watson, J. (2005). *Caring science as sacred science*. Philadelphia, PA: F. A. Davis.

Weeks, J. (2010, May 12). Reference guide: Language and sections on CAM and integrative practice in HR 3590/healthcare overhaul. *Integrator Blog*. Available at http://theintegratorblog.com/site/index .php?option=com_content&task=view&id=658&Itemid=2

White House Commission on Complementary and Alternative Medicine Policy (WHCCAMP). (2002). *Final report*. Washington, DC: U.S. Government Printing Office.

Wolf, R. (2010, September 17). Record rise in U.S. uninsured: 50.7 million. *USA Today*, p. A8.

Appendix A.

Holistic Nursing: Scope and Standards of Practice (2007)

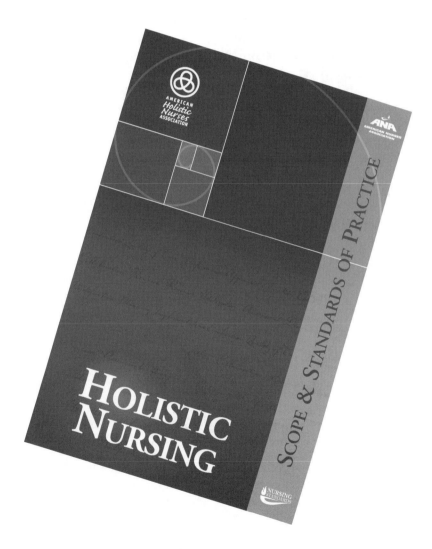

The content in this appendix is not current and is of historical significance only.

Holistic Nursing: Scope of Practice

Definition and Overview of Holistic Nursing

Holistic nursing is defined as "all nursing practice that has healing the whole person as its goal" (AHNA 1998).

Holistic nursing embraces all nursing that has the enhancement of healing the whole person from birth to death—and all age groups from infant to elder—as its goal. Holistic nursing recognizes that there are two views regarding holism: that holism involves identifying the interrelationships of the bio-psycho-social-spiritual dimensions of the person, recognizing that the whole is greater than the sum of its parts; and that holism involves understanding the individual as a unitary whole in mutual process with the environment. Holistic nursing responds to both views, believing that the goals of nursing can be achieved within either framework.

Holistic nursing focuses on protecting, promoting, and optimizing health and wellness, assisting healing, preventing illness and injury, alleviating suffering, and supporting people to find peace, comfort, harmony, and balance through the diagnosis and treatment of human response.

Holistic nursing care is person–relationship centered and healing oriented vs. disease/cure oriented. Holistic nursing emphasizes practices of self-care, intentionality, presence, mindfulness, and therapeutic use of self as pivotal for facilitation of healing and patterning of wellness in others. Holistic nursing is prospective, focusing on:

- Comprehensive health promotion and health risk reduction.

- Proactive interventions that address antecedents and mediators of disease.

- Opportunities in each individual's experiences of illness and disease for the individual's transformation, growth, and finding of meaning.

The holistic nurse is an instrument of healing and a facilitator in the healing process. Holistic nurses honor the individual's subjective experience about health, health beliefs, and values. To become therapeutic

The content in this appendix is not current and is of historical significance only.

partners with individuals, families, communities, and populations, holistic nursing practice draws on nursing knowledge, theories, research, expertise, intuition, and creativity incorporating the roles of clinician, educator, consultant, partner, role model, and advocate. Holistic nursing practice encourages peer review of professional practice in various clinical settings and provides care based on current professional standards, laws, and regulations governing nursing practice.

Holistic nurses integrate complementary/alternative modalities (CAM) into clinical practice to treat people's physiological, psychological, and spiritual needs. Doing so does not negate the validity of conventional medical therapies but serves to complement, broaden, and enrich the scope of nursing practice and to help individuals access their greatest healing potential. Integration rather than separation is advocated.

Practicing holistic nursing requires nurses to integrate self-care, self-responsibility, spirituality, and reflection in their own lives. This leads the nurse to greater awareness of the interconnectedness with oneself, others, nature, and God/LifeForce/Absolute/Transcendent. This awareness further enhances nurses' understanding of all individuals and their relationships to the human and global community, and it permits nurses to use this awareness to facilitate the healing process.

The phenomena of concern to holistic nursing include, but are not limited to:

- The caring–healing relationship
- The subjective experience of and meanings ascribed to health, illness, wellness, healing, birth, growth and development, and dying
- The cultural values and beliefs and folk practices of health, illness, and healing
- Spirituality in nursing care
- The evaluation of complementary/alternative modalities used in nursing practice
- Comprehensive health promotion and disease prevention
- Self-care processes
- Physical, mental, emotional, and spiritual comfort, discomfort, and pain

The content in this appendix is not current and is of historical significance only.

- Empowerment, decision-making, and the ability to make informed choices

- Social and economic policies and their effects on the health of individuals, families, and communities

- Diverse and alternative healthcare systems and their relationships with access and quality of health care

- The environment and the prevention of disease

This document, used in conjunction with *Nursing's Social Policy Statement, Second Edition* (ANA 2003), *Nursing: Scope and Standards of Practice* (ANA 2004), *Code of Ethics for Nurses with Interpretive Statements* (ANA 2001), and the laws, statutes, and regulations related to nursing practice for their state, commonwealth, or territory, delineates the professional responsibilities of a holistic nurse.

Evolution of Holistic Nursing

"Holism" in health care is a philosophy that emanated directly from Florence Nightingale, who believed in care that focused on unity, wellness, and the interrelationship of human beings, events, and environment. Even Hippocrates, the father of Western medicine, espoused a holistic orientation when he taught doctors to observe their patients' life circumstances and emotional states. Socrates stated, "Curing the soul; that is the first thing." In holism, symptoms are believed to be an expression of the body's wisdom as it reacts to cure its own imbalance or disease.

The root of the word *heal* comes from the Greek word *halos* and the Anglo-Saxon word *healan*, which means "to be or to become whole." The word *holy* also comes from the same source. Healing means "making whole"—or restoring balance and harmony. It is movement toward a sense of wholeness and completion. Healing therefore is the integration of the totality of the person in body, mind, emotion, spirit, and environment.

One of the driving forces behind the holistic nursing movement in the United States was the formation of the American Holistic Nurses Association (AHNA). In 1980, founder Charlotte McGuire and 75 founding members began the national organization in Houston, Texas. The national

The content in this appendix is not current and is of historical significance only.

office is now located in Flagstaff, Arizona. AHNA has as its mission to unite nurses in healing with a focus on holistic principles of health, preventive education, and the integration of allopathic and complementary caring–healing modalities to facilitate care of the whole person and significant others. From its inception in 1980, the American Holistic Nurses Association (AHNA) has been the leader in developing and advancing holistic principles, practices, and guidelines. The Association predicted that holistic principles, caring–healing, and the integration of complementary/alternative therapies would emerge into mainstream health care.

The AHNA, the definitive voice for holistic nursing, is committed to promoting wholeness and wellness in individuals/families/communities, nurses themselves, the nursing profession, and the environment. Through its various activities, the AHNA provides vision, direction, and leadership in the advancement of holistic nursing; integrates the art and science of nursing in the profession; empowers holistic nursing through education, research, and standards; encourages nurses to be models of wellness; honors individual excellence in the advancement of holistic nursing; and influences policy to change the healthcare system to a more humanistic orientation.

The goals and endeavors of the AHNA have continued to map conceptual frameworks and the blueprint for holistic nursing practice, education, and research, which is the most complete way to conceptualize and practice professional nursing. Beginning in 1993, AHNA undertook an organization development process that included the following areas:

- Identification of the steps toward national certification in 1993–1994

- Revision of the 1990 *Standards of Holistic Nursing Practice*, completed in 1995

- Completing a role delineation study, the *Inventory of Professional Activities and Knowledge Statements of a Holistic Nurse* (also known as the IPAKHN Survey) in 1997

- Developing a national Holistic Nursing Certification Examination, completed in 1997

- Completing major revisions of the 1995 *Standards of Holistic Nursing Practice* in 1999, with additional editorial changes in January 2000 and 2005

The content in this appendix is not current and is of historical significance only.

- Developing a Core Curriculum for basic holistic nursing based on the Basic Standards (1997)

- Approving and adopting *Standards of Advanced Holistic Nursing Practice for Graduate-Prepared Nurses* (2002, revised 2005)

- Developing a Core Curriculum for advanced holistic nursing based on the Advanced Standards (2003)

- Developing the Certification Exam for Advanced Holistic Nursing Practice by The American Holistic Nurses Certification Corporation (AHNCC) in 2004. This exam was first offered in March 2005.

- Revising the 2004 basic and advanced *Standards of Holistic Nursing Practice* to meet ANA criteria for recognition of holistic nursing as a specialty

Other AHNA activities that support and promote holistic nursing include:

- Collaborating with other organizations to strengthen the voice of nursing

- Endorsing certificate programs for nurses that have content in holistic nursing and/or complementary/alternative healing modalities

- Organizing networking groups to further holistic nursing

- Providing and approving continuing education programs featuring holistic health topics, holistic research, and holistic education

- Granting awards for holistic nursing research

- Publishing several informational, educational, research, and professional support materials

- Sponsoring the World-Wide Commemorative Moment for Florence Nightingale and Nursing

- Offering the National Student Sponsorship Initiative

There are now increasing numbers of holistic nurses who hold leadership roles as clinicians, educators, authors, and researchers in university-based schools of nursing, practice environments, nursing, and other professional organizations.

Membership in the AHNA is open to all individuals who support the mission of the organization. AHNA's philosophy is that holistic nursing is the *heart* of nursing and the *science* of holism.

The content in this appendix is not current and is of historical significance only.

Principles of Holistic Nursing

The following principles—Person, Healing/Health, Practice—underlie holistic nursing:

Person

- There is unity, totality, and connectedness of everyone and everything (body, mind, emotion, spirit, sexuality, age, environment, social/cultural, belief systems, relationships, context).

- Human beings are unique and inherently good.

- People are able to find meaning and purpose in their own life, experiences, and illness.

- All people have an innate power and capacity for self healing. Health/illness is subjectively described and determined by the view of the individual. Therefore, the person is honored in all phases of his/her healing process regardless of expectations or outcomes.

- People/persons/individuals are the recipients of holistic nursing services. These can be clients, patients, families, significant others, populations, or communities. They may be ill and within the health-care delivery system or well, moving toward personal betterment to enhance well-being.

Healing/Health

- Health and illness are natural and a part of life, learning, and movement toward change and development.

- Health is seen as balance, integration, harmony, right relationship, and the betterment of well-being, not just the absence of disease. Healing can take place without cure. The focus is on health promotion/disease prevention/health restoration/lifestyle patterns and habits, as well as symptom relief.

- Illness is considered a teacher and an opportunity for self-awareness and growth as part of the life process. Symptoms are respected as messages.

- People as active partners in the healing process are empowered when they take some control of their own lives, health, and well-being including personal choices and relationships.

The content in this appendix is not current and is of historical significance only.

- Treatment is a process that considers the root of the problem, not merely treating the obvious signs and symptoms.

Practice

- Practice is a science (critical thinking, reflection, evidence/research/ theory as underlying practice) and an art (intuition, creativity, presence, self/personal knowing as integral to practice).

- The values and ethic of holism, caring, moral insight, dignity, integrity, competence, responsibility, accountability, and legality underlie holistic nursing practice.

- There are various philosophies and paradigms of health, illness, healing, and approaches/models for the delivery of health care, both in the U.S. and in other cultures, that need to be understood and utilized.

- Older adults represent the predominant population served by nurses.

- Public policy and the healthcare delivery system influence the health and well-being of society and professional nursing.

Nursing Roles

- Using warmth, compassion, caring, authenticity, respect, trust, and relationship as instruments of healing in and of themselves, as part of the healing environment.

- Using conventional nursing interventions as well as holistic/ complementary/alternative/integrative modalities that enhance the body-mind-emotion-spirit-environment connectedness to foster healing, health, wholeness, and well-being of people.

- Collaborating and partnering with all constituencies in the health process including the person receiving care and family, community, peers, and other disciplines. Using principles and skills of co-operation, alliance, and respect and honoring the contributions of all.

- Participating in the change process to develop more caring cultures in which to practice and learn.

- Assisting nurses to nurture and heal themselves.

The content in this appendix is not current and is of historical significance only.

- Participating in activities that contribute to the improvement of communities and the environment and to the betterment of public health.

- Acting as an advocate for the rights of and equitable distribution and access to health care for all persons, especially vulnerable populations.

- Honoring the ecosystem and our relationship with and need to preserve it, as we are all connected.

Self-Care

- The nurse's self-reflection and self-assessment, self-care, healing, and personal development are necessary for service to others and growth/change in one's own well-being and understanding of one's own personal journey.

- The nurse values oneself and one's calling to holistic nursing as a life purpose.

Integrating the Art and Science of Nursing: Core Values

The art and science of holistic nursing emanates from these five core values, which are described in this section:

- Core Value 1. Holistic Philosophy, Theories, and Ethics

- Core Value 2. Holistic Caring Process

- Core Value 3. Holistic Communication, Therapeutic Environment, and Cultural Diversity

- Core Value 4. Holistic Education and Research

- Core Value 5. Holistic Nurse Self-Care

Core Value 1. Holistic Philosophy, Theories, and Ethics

Holistic nurses recognize the human health experience as a complicated, dynamic relationship of health, illness, and wellness, and they value healing as the desired outcome of the practice of nursing. Their practice is based on scientific foundations (theory, research, evidence-based practice, critical thinking, reflection) and art (relationship, communication, creativity, presence, caring).

The content in this appendix is not current and is of historical significance only.

Holistic nursing is grounded in nursing knowledge and skill and guided by nursing theory. Florence Nightingale's writings are often referenced as a significant precursor for the development of holistic nursing practice. While each holistic nurse chooses which nursing theory to apply in any individual case, the nursing theories of Jean Watson (Theory of Human Caring), Martha Rogers (the Science of Unitary Human Beings), Margaret Newman (Health as Expanding Consciousness), Madeleine Leininger (Theory of Cultural Care), Rosemarie Rizzo Parse (Theory of Human Becoming), Paterson and Zderad (Humanistic Nursing Theory), and Helen Erickson (Modeling and Role-Modeling) are most frequently used to support holistic nursing practice.

In addition to nursing theory, holistic nurses utilize other theories and perspectives of wholeness and healing that guide their practice. These scientific theories and philosophies present a worldview of connectedness, e.g., theories of consciousness; energy field theory; Carl Pribram's Holographic Universe; David Bohm's Implicate/Explicate Order; Candace Pert's psychoneuroimmunology; Rupert Sheldrake's morphogenic fields; Ken Wilbur's Spectrum of Consciousness and Integral Psychology; Pierre Tielhard de Chardin's philosophy; spirituality; and alternative medical systems such as traditional Oriental medicine, Ayurveda, Native American and indigenous healing, and Eastern contemplative orientations such as Zen and Taoism.

Holistic nurses further recognize and honor the ethic that the person is the authority on his or her own health experience. The holistic nurse is an "option giver," i.e., helping the person develop an understanding of alternatives and implications of various health and treatment options.

The holistic nurse first ascertains what the individual thinks or believes is happening to them and then assists the person to identify what will help his/her situation. The assessment begins from where the individual is. The holistic nurse then discusses options, including the person's choices, across a continuum, including possible effects and implications of each. For instance, if a person diagnosed with cancer is experiencing nausea due to chemotherapy, the individual and nurse may discuss the choices and effects of pharmacologic agents, imagery, homeopathic remedies, etc., or a combination of these. The holistic nurse acts as partner and co-prescriptor vs. sole prescriber. The relationship is a co-piloting of the individual's health experience in which the nurse respects

The content in this appendix is not current and is of historical significance only.

the person's decision about his or her own health. It is a process of engagement rather than compliance.

Client narratives, whether they arise from individuals, families, or communities, provide the context of the experiences and are used as an important focus in understanding the person's situation. Holistic nurses hold the belief that people, through their inherent capacities, heal themselves. Therefore, the holistic nurse is not the healer but the guide and facilitator of the individual's own healing.

In the belief that all things are connected, the holistic perspective espouses that an individual's actions have a ripple effect throughout humanity. Holism places the greatest worth on individuals' developing higher levels of human awareness. This, in turn, elevates the whole of humanity. Holistic nurses believe in the sacredness of one's self and of all nature. One's inner self and the collective greater self have stewardship not only over one's body, mind, and spirit, but also over our planet. Holistic nurses focus on the meaning and quality of life deriving from their own character and from their relationship to the universe rather than imposed from without.

Holistic nurses hold to a professional ethic of caring and healing that seeks to preserve wholeness and dignity of self and others. They support human dignity by advocating and adhering to *The Patient's Bill of Rights in Medicare and Medicaid* (U.S. DHHS 1999a), ANA's *Code of Ethics for Nurses with Interpretive Standards* (2001), and AHNA's *Position Statement on Holistic Nursing Ethics* (2007), the latter of which is included in Appendix D (page 120).

Core Value 2. Holistic Caring Process

Holistic nurses provide care that recognizes the totality of the human being (the interconnectedness of body, mind, emotion, spirit, social/cultural, relationship, context, and environment). This is an integrated as well as comprehensive approach. While physical symptoms are being treated, a holistic nurse would also focus on how the individual is cognitively perceiving and emotionally dealing with the illness; its effect on the person's family and social relationships and economic resources; the person's values and cultural, spiritual beliefs and preferences regarding treatment; and the meaning of this experience to the person's life. But in addition, a holistic nurse may also incorporate a number of

The content in this appendix is not current and is of historical significance only.

alternative modalities (e.g., cognitive restructuring, stress management, visualization and imagery, hypnotherapy, aromatherapy, Therapeutic Touch, Healing Touch) with conventional nursing interventions. Holistic nurses focus on care interventions that promote healing, peace, comfort, and a subjective sense of well-being for the person.

The holistic caring process involves six often simultaneously occurring steps: assessment, diagnosis (identification of pattern/problem/need/health issue), outcomes, therapeutic plan of care, implementation, and evaluation. Holistic nurses apply the holistic caring process with individuals or families across the lifespan, population groups, and communities, and in all settings.

Holistic nurses incorporate a variety of roles in their practice, including expert clinician and facilitator of healing; consultant and collaborator; educator and guide; administrator, leader, and change agent; researcher; and advocate. They strongly emphasize partnership with individuals throughout the entire decision-making process.

Holistic assessments include not only the physical, functional, psychosocial, mental, emotional, cultural, and sexual aspects, but also the spiritual, transpersonal, and energy field assessments of the whole person. Energy assessments are based on the concept that all beings are composed of energy. Congestion or stagnation of energy in any realm creates dis-harmony and dis-ease. Spiritual assessments glean not only religious beliefs and practices but also query about a person's meaning and purpose in life and how that may have changed due to the present health experience. Spiritual assessments also include questions about an individual's sense of serenity and peace, what provides joy and fulfillment, and the source of strength and hope.

Holistic assessment data are interpreted into patterns/challenges/needs from which meaning and understanding of the health/disease experience can be mutually identified with the person. An important responsibility is that of helping the person to identify risk factors such as lifestyle, habits, beliefs and values, personal and family health history, and age-related conditions that influence health and then to utilize opportunities to increase well-being. The focus is on the individual's goals, not the nurse's goals.

Therapeutic plans of care respect the person's experience and the uniqueness of each healing journey. The same illness may have very

The content in this appendix is not current and is of historical significance only.

different manifestations in different individuals. A major aspect of holistic nursing practice, in addition to competence, is intention—that is, intending for the wholeness, well-being, and highest good of the person with every encounter and intervention. This honors and reinforces the innate capacity of people to heal themselves. Therefore, holistic nurses respect that outcomes may not be those expected and may evolve differently based on the person's own individual healing process and health choices. Holistic nurses endeavor to detach themselves from the outcomes. The nurse does not produce the outcomes; the individual's own healing process produces the outcomes, and the nurse facilitates this process. A significant focus is on guiding individuals and significant others to utilize their own inner strength and resources through the course of healing.

Appropriate and evidence-based information (including current knowledge, practice, and research) regarding the health condition and various treatments and therapies and their side effects is consistently provided. Holistic care always occurs within the scope and standards of practice of registered nursing and in accordance with state and federal laws and regulations.

In addition to conventional interventions, holistic nurses have knowledge of and integrate a number of CAM approaches, which have been categorized by the National Center for Complementary and Alternative Medicine (2005). (See also Appendix A.) These include the following categories:

- Whole medical systems, such as Ayurveda, Traditional Oriental Medicine, Homeopathy, Naturopathy, Acupuncture, Native American and Latin American indigenous practices

- Mind–body interventions, such as meditation, relaxation, imagery, hypnosis, yoga, t'ai chi, prayer, art, music and dance therapies, cognitive-behavioral therapy, biofeedback, therapeutic counseling, and stress management

- Biologically based therapies, such as herbal therapies, diet therapies, nutritional supplements, and vitamin and mineral supplements

- Manipulative and body-based methods, such as chiropractic, massage therapy, osteopathy, Rolfing, reflexology, Alexander Technique, and Craniosacral therapy

- Energy therapies, such as Therapeutic Touch, Reiki, Qi Gong, Acupressure, Healing Touch, and magnet therapy

Therapies frequently incorporated in holistic nursing practice include the following interventions listed in the Nursing Interventions Classification (NIC): meditation; relaxation therapy; breath work; music, art, aroma therapies; energy-based touch therapies such as Therapeutic Touch, Healing Touch, Reiki; acupressure; massage; guided imagery; animal-assisted therapy; biofeedback; prayer; reflexology; diet; herbology; and homeopathy. Interventions frequently employed in holistic nursing practice in addition to conventional nursing interventions include: anxiety reduction and stress management, calming technique, emotional support, exercise and nutrition promotion, smoking cessation promotion, patient contracting, resiliency promotion, forgiveness facilitation, hope installation, presence, journaling, counseling, cognitive therapy, self-help, spiritual support, and environmental management.

As many of today's healthcare problems are stress related, holistic nurses empower individuals by teaching them techniques to reduce their stress. Many interventions used in holistic nursing elicit the relaxation response (e.g., breath work, meditation, relaxation, imagery, aromatherapy and use of essential oils, diet). People can learn these therapies and use them without the intervention of a healthcare provider. This allows a person to take an active role in the management of his/her own health care. Holistic nurses also can teach families and caregivers to use these techniques for loved ones who may be ill (e.g., simple foot or hand massage for older clients with dementia). In addition, individuals are taught how to evaluate their own responses to these modalities.

Holistic nurses prescribe as legally authorized. They instruct individuals regarding drug, herbal, and homeopathic regimens and, importantly, the side effects and interactions of these therapies. They consult, collaborate, and refer, as necessary, to both conventional allopathic providers and to holistic practitioners. They provide information and counseling to people about alternative, complementary, integrative, and conventional healthcare practices. Very importantly, holistic nurses facilitate negotiation of services as they guide individuals and families between conventional Western medical and alternative systems. Holistic nurses, in partnership with the individual and others, evaluate if care is effective and if there are changes in the meaning of the health experience for the individual.

Core Value 3. Holistic Communication, Therapeutic Environment, and Cultural Diversity

The holistic nurse's communication ensures that each individual experiences the presence of the nurse as authentic, caring, compassionate, and sincere. This is more than simply using therapeutic techniques such as responding, reflecting, summarizing, etc. This is deep listening or, as some say, "listening with the heart and not just the ears." It is done with conscious intention and without preconceptions, busyness, distractions, or analysis. It takes place in the "now" within an atmosphere of shared humanness, i.e., human being to human being. Through presence or "being with in the moment," holistic nurses provide each person with an interpersonal encounter that is experienced as a connection with one who is giving *undivided* attention to the needs and concerns of the individual. Using unconditional positive regard, holistic nurses convey to the individual receiving care the belief in his or her worth and value as a human being, not solely the recipient of medical and nursing interventions.

The importance of context in understanding the person's health experience is always recognized. Space and time are allowed for exploration. Each person's health encounter is truly seen as unique and may be contrary to conventional knowledge and treatments. Therefore, the holistic nurse must be comfortable with ambiguity, paradox, and uncertainty. This requires a perspective that the nurse is not "the expert" regarding another's health/illness experience.

Holistic nurses have a knowledge base of the use and meanings of symbolic language and use interventions such as imagery, creation of sacred space and personal rituals, dream exploration, and aesthetic therapies such as music, visual arts, and dance. They encourage and support others in the use of prayer, meditation, or other spiritual and symbolic practices for healing purposes.

A cornerstone of holistic nursing practice is assisting individuals to find meaning in their experience. Regardless of the health/illness condition, the meaning that individuals ascribe to their situation can influence their response to it. Holistic nurses attend to the subjective world of the individual. They consider meanings such as the person's concerns in relation to health, family relationships, employment, and economics, as well as to deeper meanings related to the person's purpose in life. Regardless of the technology or treatment, holistic nurses address the

The content in this appendix is not current and is of historical significance only.

human spirit as a major force in healing. The person's perception of meaning is related to all factors in health-wellness-disease-illness.

Holistic nurses realize that suffering, illness, and disease are natural components of the human condition and have the potential to teach about oneself, one's relationships, and the universe. Every experience is valued for its meaning and lesson.

Holistic nurses have a particular obligation to create a therapeutic environment that values holism, caring, social support, and integration of conventional and CAM approaches to healing. They seek to create caring cultures and environments where individuals, both clients and staff, feel connected, supported, and respected. A particular perspective of holistic nursing is the nurse as the "healing environment" and an instrument of healing. Holistic nurses shape the physical environment (e.g., light, fresh air, pleasant sounds or quiet, neatness and order, healing smells, earth elements). They also provide a relationship-focused environment, the creation of sacred space through presence and intention where others can feel safe, can unfold, can explore the dimensions of self in healing.

Culture, beliefs, and values are an inherent component of a holistic approach. Concepts of health and healing are based in culture and often influence people's actions to promote, maintain, and restore health. Culture also may provide an understanding of a person's concept of the illness or disease and appropriate treatment. Holistic nurses possess knowledge and understanding of numerous cultural traditions and healthcare practices from various racial, ethnic, and social backgrounds. However, holistic nurses honor individuals' understanding and articulation of their own cultural values, beliefs, and health practices rather than reliance on stereotypical cultural classifications and descriptions. These understandings then are used to provide culturally competent care that corresponds with the beliefs, values, traditions, and health practices of individuals and families. Holistic nurses ask individuals, "What do I need to know about you culturally in caring for you?"

Holistic healing is a collaborative approach. Holistic nurses take an active role in trying to remove the political and financial barriers to the inclusion of holistic care in the healthcare system.

Of particular importance to holistic nurses is the human connection with the ecology. They actively participate in building an ecosystem that

The content in this appendix is not current and is of historical significance only.

sustains the well-being of all life. This includes raising the public's consciousness about environmental issues and stressors that affect not only the health of people, but also the health of the planet.

Core Value 4. Holistic Education and Research

Holistic nurses possess an understanding of a wide range of cultural norms and healthcare practices/beliefs/values concerning individuals, families, groups, and communities from varied racial ethnic, spiritual, and social backgrounds. This rich knowledge base reflects their formal academic and continuing education preparation and also includes a wide diversity of practices and modalities outside of conventional medicine. Because of this preparation, holistic nurses serve as both educators and advocates and have a significant impact on peoples' understanding of healthcare options and alternatives.

Additionally, holistic nurses provide much-needed information to individuals on health promotion including such topics as healthy lifestyles, risk-reducing behaviors, preventive self-care, stress management, living with changes secondary to illness and treatment, and opportunities to enhance well-being.

Holistic nurses value all the ways of knowing and learning. They individualize learning and appreciate that science, intuition, introspection, creativity, aesthetics, and culture produce different bodies of knowledge and perspectives. They help others to know themselves and access their own inner wisdom to enhance growth, wholeness, and well-being.

Holistic nurses often guide individuals and families in their healthcare decisions, especially regarding conventional allopathic and complementary alternative practices. Therefore, they must be knowledgeable about the best evidence available for both conventional and CAM therapies. In addition to developing evidence-based practice using research, practice guidelines, and expertise, holistic nurses strongly consider the person's values and healthcare practices and beliefs in practice decisions.

Holistic nurses look at alternative philosophies of science and research methods that are compatible with investigations of humanistic and holistic occurrences; that explore the context in which phenomena occur and the meaning of patterns that evolve; and that take into consideration the interactive nature of the body, mind, emotion, spirit, and environment.

The content in this appendix is not current and is of historical significance only.

Holistic nurses conduct and evaluate research in diverse areas such as:

- Outcome measures of various holistic therapies, e.g., Therapeutic Touch, prayer, aromatherapy

- Instrument development to measure caring behaviors and dimensions; spirituality; self-transcendence; cultural competence, etc.

- Client responses to holistic interventions in health/illness

- Explorations of clients' lived experiences with various health/illness phenomena

- Theory development in healing, caring, intentionality, cultural constructions, empowerment, etc.

Core Value 5. Holistic Nurse Self-Care

Self-care as well as personal awareness of and continuous focus on being an instrument of healing are significant requirements for holistic nurses. Holistic nurses value themselves and mobilize the necessary resources to care for themselves. They endeavor to integrate self-awareness, self-care, and self-healing into their lives by incorporating practices such as self-assessment, meditation, yoga, good nutrition, energy therapies, movement, art, support, and lifelong learning. Holistic nurses honor their unique patterns and the development of the body, the psychological-social-cultural self, the intellectual self, and the spiritual self. Nurses cannot facilitate healing unless they are in the process of healing themselves. Through continuing education, practice, and self-work, holistic nurses develop the skills of authentic and deep self-reflection and introspection to understand themselves and their journey. It is seen as a lifelong process.

Holistic nurses strive to achieve harmony/balance in their own lives and assist others to do the same. They create healing environments for themselves by attending to their own well-being, letting go of self-destructive behaviors and attitudes, and practicing centering and stress reduction techniques. By doing this, holistic nurses serve as role models to others, be they clients, colleagues, or personal contacts.

Settings for Holistic Nursing Practice

Holistic nurses practice in numerous settings, including but not limited to: private practitioner offices; ambulatory, acute, long-term, and home care settings; complementary care centers; women's health centers; hospice palliative care; psychiatric mental health facilities; schools; rehabilitation centers; community nursing organizations; student and employee health clinics; managed care organizations; independent self-employed practice; correctional facilities; professional nursing and healthcare organizations; administration; staff development; and universities and colleges.

Holistic nursing practice also occurs when there is a request for consultation or when holistic nurses advocate for care that promotes health and prevents disease, illness, or disability for individuals, communities, or the environment, e.g., a holistic nurse may choose not to work in a critical care setting but provide consultation regarding self-care or stress management to nurses in that area. Or, holistic nurses may practice in preoperative and recovery rooms instituting a "Prepare for Surgery" program that teaches individuals having surgery meditation and positive affirmation techniques, pre and post surgery, while incorporating a homeopathic regimen for trauma and cell healing. Employment or voluntary participation of holistic nurses also can influence civic activities and the regulatory and legislative arena at the local, state, national, or international level.

As holistic nursing focuses on wellness, wholeness, and development of the whole person, holistic nurses also practice in health enhancement settings such as spas, gyms, and wellness centers.

Because holistic nursing is a worldview, a way of "being" in the world and not just a modality, holistic nurses can practice in any setting and with individuals throughout the life span. As the public increasingly requests holistic/CAM services, holistic nurses will be increasingly in demand and practice in a wider array of settings. Holistic nursing takes place wherever healing occurs.

Educational Preparation for Holistic Nursing

Holistic nurses are registered nurses who are educationally prepared for practice from an approved school of nursing and are licensed to practice in their individual state, commonwealth, or territory. The holistic registered nurse's experience, education, knowledge, and abilities establish the level of competence. This document identifies the scope of prac-

The content in this appendix is not current and is of historical significance only.

tice of holistic nursing and the specific standards and associated measurement criteria of holistic nurses at both the basic and advanced levels. Regardless of the level of practice, all holistic nurses integrate the previously identified five core values.

A registered nurse may prepare for the specialty of holistic nursing in a variety of ways. Educational offerings range from baccalaureate and graduate courses and programs to continuing education programs with extensive contact hours.

Basic Practice Level

The education of all nursing students preparing for RN licensure includes basic content on physiological, psychological, emotional, and some spiritual processes with populations across the life span and conventional nursing care practices within each of these domains. Additionally, basic nursing education incorporates experiences in a variety of clinical/practice settings from acute care to community. However, the educational focus is most frequently on "specialties" often emanating from the biomedical disease model with cure orientation.

In holistic nursing, the individual across the life span is viewed in context as an integrated body, mind, emotion, social, spirit totality, with the emphasis on wholeness, well-being, health promotion, and healing using both conventional and complementary/alternative practices. Because of the lack of intentional focus on integration, unity, and healing, the educational exposure of most nursing students is not adequate preparation for assuming the specialty role of a holistic nurse.

There are currently seven undergraduate programs in the U.S. endorsed by the American Holistic Nurse Certification Corporation (AHNCC) that prepare undergraduate students in holistic nursing. Additionally, there are many schools of nursing offering both graduate and undergraduate courses in "Holistic Nursing." A survey of schools of nursing in the United States (Fenton and Morris 2003) indicated that almost 60% (n=74) of the responding schools (sample n=125 schools) had a definition of holistic nursing in their curricula and were familiar with *Holistic Nursing Core Curriculum* (see Dossey 1997). The majority of the sample (84.8%, n=106) included at least one complementary/alternative modality (e.g., visualization, relaxation) in their curricula. Twenty-six (21%) schools had faculty who were certified in holistic nursing.

The content in this appendix is not current and is of historical significance only.

Increasingly, schools of nursing are incorporating holistic nursing practices and complementary/alternative modalities into their curricula, responding to consumer use of CAM and consumer demand for health professionals who are knowledgeable about holistic practices.

To be board certified by the AHNCC at the basic holistic nursing level, a nurse is required to have: (1) an active, unrestricted U.S. license; (2) a baccalaureate or higher degree; (3) at least one year of full-time practice or 2,000 hours of part-time practice within the last five years as a holistic nurse or graduation from an AHNCC-endorsed university; (4) a minimum of 48 contact hours of holistic nursing continuing education within the last 2 years.

Advanced Practice Level

As with the basic level, there are a variety of ways (both academic and professional development) in which registered nurses can acquire the additional specialized knowledge and skills that prepare them for practice as an advanced practice holistic nurse. These nurses are expected to have an active, unrestricted U.S. license and to hold a master's or doctoral degree in nursing and demonstrate a greater depth and scope of knowledge, a greater integration of information, increased complexity of skills and interventions, and notable role autonomy. They provide leadership in practice, teaching, research, consultation, advocacy, and/or policy formation in advancing holistic nursing to improve the holistic health of people.

Presently five graduate programs in the United States that prepare master's students with a specialty in holistic nursing are endorsed by the AHNCC. Other graduate nursing programs have courses in holistic or complementary/alternative practices. Current advanced practice nurses (nurse practitioners, clinical nurse specialists, nurse midwives, nurse anesthetists) are increasingly gaining specialized knowledge preparing them as holistic nurses through post-master's degree programs, continuing education offerings, and certificate programs.

To be board certified by the AHNCC at the advanced holistic nursing level, a licensed nurse must have a graduate degree in nursing and a minimum of 48 contact hours in holistic nursing within the last 2 years.

Continuing Education for Basic and Advanced Practice Levels

The American Holistic Nurses Association (AHNA) is a provider and approver of continuing education, recognized by the American Nurses Credentialing Center. Continuing educational programs, workshops, and lectures in holistic nursing and CAM have been popular nationwide, with AHNA or other bodies granting continuing education units.

AHNA endorses certificate programs in specific areas, including Spirituality, Health and Healing, Reflexology, Imagery, Aromatherapy, Healing Touch, AMMA Therapy®, Clinical Nursing Assessment, and Whole Health Education. It also approves continuing education offerings in holistic nursing and offers the AHNA home study course, Foundations of Holistic Nursing. Other programs in distinct therapies such as Acupuncture, Reiki, Homeopathy, massage, imagery, healing arts, holistic health, Oriental Medicine, nutrition, Ayurveda, Therapeutic Touch, Healing Touch, herbology, chiropractic, etc. are given nationally as degrees, certificates, or continuing education programs by centers, specialty organizations, or schools.

Certification in Holistic Nursing

In 1992, a four-phase AHNA Certificate Program in Holistic Nursing began. On program completion, a nurse was awarded a certificate in holistic nursing. In 1994, the AHNA Leadership Council appointed an AHNA Task Force Committee to explore steps toward the development of holistic nursing certification through a national certification examination.

The AHNA Leadership Council appointed an AHNA Certification Committee to serve as the governing body to oversee the process of certification of holistic nurses by examination until a separate certification corporation was established. In 1997, the AHNA Certification Board established a separate 501C-3 organization, the American Holistic Nurses' Certification Corporation (AHNCC), to act as the credentialing body for the Holistic Nursing Certification Examination. The AHNCC now has five directors who are voting members, and two non-voting members, one of whom is the liaison of the AHNA Leadership Council. Of the voting members, one represents the public and need not be an RN. All the Directors who serve on the AHNCC have been chosen for their skill in and knowledge of holistic nursing and of the process of certification. There is a public member who is not a registered nurse.

The content in this appendix is not current and is of historical significance only.

The AHNCC is an autonomous body with administrative independence in matters pertaining to specialty certification. The AHNCC maintains a collaborative relationship with but is not involved with the AHNA continuing education, endorsement, or accreditation activities.

The AHNCC defines certification as a qualifying process attesting that an individual, who is already practicing as a registered nurse and demonstrating basic nursing competencies, has met predetermined criteria for basic or advanced specialized practice. In relation to holistic nursing certification, the nurse must demonstrate competencies of specialized nursing practice encompassing holism.

The purpose of a certification process is to provide nurses with a standard they can be measured against, and to be able to declare to the community at large that certain individuals are competent to practice holistic nursing.

AHNCC National Board Certification in holistic nursing is available at the basic (HN-BC) level, which requires a baccalaureate degree, and advanced (AHN-BC) level, which requires a graduate degree. The process for basic certification includes a formal qualitative review of an applicant's portfolio documenting the practice of holistic nursing (RN licensure, academic credentials, holistic nursing experience, continuing education, or successful completion of the certificate program in holistic nursing), and a quantitative certification exam that was developed jointly by the AHNA and the National League of Nursing testing office. The Advanced Certification Exam was developed jointly by the AHNCC and the Professional Testing Service and first offered in March 2005. The process for advanced level certification also requires a qualitative assessment and a quantitative advanced certification exam. Recertification for both basic and advanced levels is completed by documentation of contact hours in holistic nursing.

Further, the AHNCC provides endorsement for university-based undergraduate and graduate nursing programs whose curricula meet the holistic nursing standards in this book (*Holistic Nursing: Scope and Standards of Practice*) so their graduates may sit for the certification exam without providing a qualitative assessment.

Continued Commitment to the Profession

The specialty practice of holistic nursing is generally not well understood. Therefore each holistic nurse must educate other nurses, health-

The content in this appendix is not current and is of historical significance only.

care providers, professionals, and the public about the role, value, and benefits of holistic nursing, whether it be in direct practice, education, management, or research. Holistic nurses articulate the ideas of the holistic paradigm and the philosophy of the caring–healing model. Jean Watson reminds us that society and the public are searching for something deeper in terms of realizing self-care, self-knowledge, and self-healing potentials. Nurses need to acknowledge the human aspects of practice, attending to people and their experience rather than just focusing on the medical orientation and disease. She concludes that "nurses have a covenant with the public to sustain caring. It is our collective responsibility to transform caring practices into the framework that identifies and gives distinction to nursing as a profession" (Watson 2005, p. 12).

Holistic nurses are committed to continuous, lifelong learning and personal growth for self and others. As role models, they engage in self-assessment and commit to practicing self-care to enhance their physical, psychological, intellectual, social, and spiritual well-being.

Holistic nurses promote the advancement of the profession and holistic nursing by participating in professional and community organizations, writing, publishing, and speaking to professional and lay or public audiences. By engaging in local, state, national, and international forums, they strive to increase the awareness of holistic health issues and the development of holistic care models.

Holistic nurses are particularly attentive to their role as advocates for both people and the environment. They seek to understand the political, social, ethnic, organizational, financial, and discriminatory barriers to holistic care for individuals, population groups, and communities. Holistic nurses work to eliminate these barriers, particularly for the repressed and underserved. They respect and honor people's dignity and freedom to choose among existing alternatives. Holistic nurses assist and empower people to develop self-advocacy skills and make educated life choices. Holistic nurses engage in activities that respect, nurture, and enhance the integral relationship with the earth, contributing to creating an ecosystem that supports the well-being of all life. Acting as teachers, leaders, collaborators, and consultants, they evaluate global health issues and environmental safety, and assist in reducing or eliminating the effects of environmental hazards on the health or welfare of individuals, groups, and communities.

The content in this appendix is not current and is of historical significance only.

Care of Older Adults

Holistic nursing care is provided to people of all ages across the continuum of care from health promotion and wellness care to acute illness care. Holistic nursing recognizes that older adults represent the predominant population in the healthcare delivery system, a unique population who can benefit greatly from holistic nursing services. Currently, there are more than 36 million people ages 65 or older in the U.S., and this number will increase dramatically by 2011 when many of the baby boomers turn 65. Aging is a multidimensional experience that encompasses the interrelatedness of the body-mind-emotion-spirit-environment. It includes physical, sensory, affective, cognitive, behavioral, sociocultural, and spiritual elements. As aging is a holistic experience, the elderly must be approached in an individualized and comprehensive manner.

As a result of advances in health care during the past century, nurses are caring less frequently for people dying from infections and accidents, major sources of mortality at the turn of the century. Today nurses are often caring for older adults with chronic illnesses, which are a significant source of morbidity and mortality. Older adults dying of infectious processes tend to do so as a result of complications of a chronic illness or debilitation. These chronic conditions contribute significantly to increased healthcare costs. Most of these leading causes of disability and death in the United States are modifiable, and in some cases are preventable. In addition, despite an increased incidence of disease and disability, poor health is not an inevitable consequence of aging.

Adopting healthy lifestyles—getting regular physical exercise, having social support, maintaining a healthy diet, avoiding tobacco and substance use, and receiving regular health-care screenings (e.g., for breast, cervical, and colorectal cancers, for diabetes, and for depression)—can dramatically reduce a person's risk of chronic illnesses.

Not only do a majority of elders experience a chronic condition, but most also have to live with and manage several chronic conditions concurrently. Adopting better lifestyle habits, in conjunction with many of the complementary modalities available to older adults, offers tremendous potential in improving quality of life for older adults, as well as decreasing co-morbidities (e.g., immobility, pain, dementia) associated with chronic illnesses. Many chronic conditions could be aided by a holistic approach and a variety of CAM therapies.

The content in this appendix is not current and is of historical significance only.

The 1999 National Health Interview Study (U.S. DHHS 1999b) indicated that CAM use increases with age (39% for age 50-plus and 70% for age 85 years and older). Older adults use CAM therapies to treat these common problems:

- Back pain or problems

- Neck pain or problems

- Joint pain or stiffness

- Anxiety

- Depression

Most users of CAM therapies do so without the knowledge or guidance of any healthcare professional. This certainly can pose a risk in geriatric care in that older adults may be:

- Self-diagnosing and self-treating with CAM products and therapies that could delay the diagnosis and perhaps more appropriate treatment for a health condition

- Unknowingly subjecting themselves to complications associated with interactions or adverse reactions to CAM therapies

- Wasting limited funds on CAM products and services that are ineffective for their specific conditions

Nurses can make a critical difference in assuring that older adults receive maximum benefit at minimum risk as they integrate CAM and conventional therapies.

Elders benefit by using holistic CAM therapies because:

- Holistic therapies build on the body's capabilities and are aimed toward strengthening the body's own defenses and healing abilities so that it can do for itself. Strengthened and healthy defenses offer elders benefits that exceed symptom management.

- Total health state is considered and a balanced lifestyle is promoted to control existing health problems, prevent new problems, and enhance general health state.

- Holistic therapies view the person holistically, realizing that people are complex combinations of unique bodies, minds, emotions, and

The content in this appendix is not current and is of historical significance only.

spirits. CAM considers this interconnectedness as it assesses and addresses the physical, mental, emotional, environmental, and spiritual aspects of the person.

- Healing practices are tailored to the individual. This is especially true for older adults, each of whom is the product of an individualized aging process. Whole-person practices offer customized healing measures.

- Holistic therapies empower older adults and encourage self-care. People are taught about self-care practices, guided in using them, and assisted in exploring possible obstacles. Older adults are empowered when they are encouraged to take maximum responsibility for their care. Also, family members and caregivers can be taught simple holistic techniques to use with their loved ones and themselves, thereby empowering the caregivers/family to participate in the elder's care and reduce their own stress.

- The elder is honored by receiving the attention needed. The abbreviated office visit, common in conventional practice, causes many elders to feel that they must be selective in what they share with their healthcare provider. As a result, questions, emotional problems, socioeconomic concerns, and spiritual issues that affect health may not be shared. In contrast, holistic practitioners are more likely to spend time learning about the total person and address needs holistically.

- Most holistic therapies are safer and gentler than conventional therapies. A variety of age-related changes, combined with the high volume and nature of medications used, cause drugs to carry many risks for elders. Although there are conditions for which drugs provide remarkable benefit, there are other conditions that can be managed and improved through lower-risk CAM approaches.

(Adapted from Eliopoulos 2005 and Shelky 2005.)

With the many benefits that can be derived from using CAM and a holistic approach, holistic nurses can best assist elders by helping them to integrate CAM with conventional therapies. This requires that nurses understand the intended and safe use of various CAM therapies, educate elders in appropriate CAM use, and prepare themselves to offer selected CAM therapies as part of their practice.

The content in this appendix is not current and is of historical significance only.

As part of its continued commitment to improve the quality of health care for older adults and advanced geriatric competence in holistic nursing practice, the AHNA offers a series of continuing education modules on topics related to Geriatric Nursing. These modules were developed through a grant (Nurse Competency in Aging Grant) from the ANA and the John A. Hartford Foundation Institute for Geriatric Nursing, New York University.

AHNA is disseminating the message that competency in geriatric care is relevant for all nurses as the demographics of the population rapidly shift. The AHNA is dedicated to making geriatric care an integral part of holistic nursing education. Additionally, AHNA has launched a geriatric nursing resource on its website for information about caring for older adults as part of holistic nursing practice (www.ahna.org/new/GeroFocus.html).

Current Trends and Issues

(The material in this section has been adapted with permission of Springer Publications from Mariano 2003.)

Trends in Holistic Nursing

The American public is increasingly demanding health care that is compassionate, respectful, provides options, is economically feasible, and is grounded in holistic ideals. A shift is occurring in health care where people desire to be more actively involved in health decision-making. They have expressed their dissatisfaction with conventional (Western) medicine and are calling for a care system that encompasses health, quality of life, and relationship with their providers (Barnes et al. 2004). The American public has pursued alternative and complementary care at an ever-increasing rate. In 1993 David Eisenberg and colleagues published a now-classic study that indicated that one-third (61 million) of Americans were using some form of alternative or complementary form of medicine (Eisenberg et al. 1993). Their continued study on use of complementary/alternative care in 1998 indicated that the use of such modalities not only continued, but sharply increased to 42% (83 million Americans). The total number of visits to providers of complementary care increased by 47%, from 427 million in 1990 to 629 million in 1997 (Eisenberg et al. 1998).

The content in this appendix is not current and is of historical significance only.

The out-of-pocket dollars spent on complementary/alternative modalities by the American public was $12.2 billion, which exceeded the out-of-pocket expenditures for all U.S. hospitalizations and compared with total out-of-pocket expense for all physician services. The most recent surveys (Barnes et al. 2004 and IOM 2005) indicate that 62% of the American public used some form of complementary/alternative modalities during the previous 12 months and estimate that between $36 to $47 billion was spent on CAM therapies.

A July 2006 survey by Health Forum, a subsidiary of the American Hospital Association (AHA), indicated that 27% of surveyed hospitals (N=1,400) are offering CAM programs to their patients. The reasons cited for offering CAM services are patient demand, clinical effectiveness, desire to treat the "whole person—body, mind, and spirit," attracting new patients, and providing additional services to existing patients.

Western medicine is proving wholly or partially ineffective for a significant proportion of common chronic diseases. Furthermore, highly technological healthcare is too expensive to be universally affordable. Holistic care that promotes health is more cost-effective and culturally acceptable to diverse and disparate populations whose belief systems are more congruent with whole-system and holistic approaches to treatment. The use of alternative methods for economic and cultural reasons by such populations often outweighs their use of conventional treatments.

An issue of CDC's *Advance Data from Vital and Health Statistics* on CAM use in the United States (Barnes et al. 2004) noted characteristics commonly associated with CAM therapies: "Individualized diagnosis and treatment of patients; an emphasis on maximizing the body's inherent healing ability; and treatment of the 'whole' person by addressing their physical, mental, and spiritual attributes rather than focusing on a specific pathogenic process as emphasized in conventional medicine" (p. 2). The National Center for Complementary and Alternative Medicine *Strategic Plan for 2005–2009* (NCCAM 2005) and *Healthy People 2010 Midcourse Review* (U.S. DHHS 2005) have set as priorities enhancing physical and mental health and wellness, preventing disease, and empowering the public to take responsibility for their health.

The White House Commission on CAM Policy (WHCCAMP) *Final Report* (2002) stated that people have come to recognize that a healthy lifestyle can promote wellness and prevent illness and disease, and

The content in this appendix is not current and is of historical significance only.

many individuals have used CAM modalities to attain this goal. Wellness incorporates a broad array of activities and interventions that focus on the physical, mental, spiritual, and emotional aspects of one's life. The effectiveness of the healthcare delivery system in the future will depend on its ability to use all approaches and modalities to contribute to a sound base for promoting health. Early interventions that promote the development of good health habits and attitudes could help modify many of the negative behaviors and lifestyle choices that began in adolescence and continue into old age. The report recommends that:

- more evidence-based teaching about CAM approaches is included in the conventional health professional schools;

- emphasis on the importance of approaches to prevent disease and promote wellness for long-term health of the American people;

- the teaching of the principles and practices of self-care and lifestyle counseling in professional schools be increased in importance, so that health professionals can, in turn, provide this guidance to their patients as well as to improve practitioners' health;

- those in the greatest need, including the chronically ill and those with limited incomes, must have available the most accurate, up-to-date information about which therapies and products may help and which may harm; and

- the education and training of all practitioners should be designed to increase the availability of practitioners knowledgeable in both CAM and conventional practices.

Weeks (2001) outlined several trends in holistic therapies that demonstrate how consumer use is influencing insurance coverage, education, and practice:

- The majority of physicians support the use of at least one or more CAM therapies.

- Approximately two-thirds of health maintenance organizations offered some coverage for CAM services, and that trend is increasing.

- The American Hospital Association has developed a program to educate member institutions on how to offer CAM services.

- Agencies such as Agency for Health Research and Quality, Bureau of Primary Health Care, Center for Disease Control and Prevention

The content in this appendix is not current and is of historical significance only.

(CDC), Health Care Financing Administration (HCFA), and the Veterans Administration have explored CAM's role in their service delivery systems.

- Integrative clinics that include both CAM and conventional providers are increasing across the country.

This driving force will propel mainstream health care increasingly in this direction, and holistic nurses are in a prime position to meet this need and provide leadership in this national trend.

In the last five to seven years, many conventional healthcare institutions have developed programs, including stress management, energy therapies, healers in the operating rooms, and acupuncture. Programs such as Reiki or Therapeutic Touch for chronic pain, support groups using imagery for breast cancer, and groups espousing meditation for health and wellness are commonly advertised across the United States. Similarly, local pharmacies and health food stores are selling an array of supplements, herbs, homeopathic preparations, vitamins, hormones, and various combinations of these that were not considered marketable five years ago. The number of books, journals, and Web sites devoted to complementary, integrative, and holistic healing practices has also dramatically increased.

Having healthcare providers who have knowledge and skill in promotion of healthful living and integration of complementary/alternative modalities is a critical need for Americans (IOM 2005). Holistic nurses are professionals who have knowledge of a wide range of complementary/alternative/integrative modalities; health promotion/restoration and disease prevention strategies; and relationship-centered, caring ways of healing.

Issues in Holistic Nursing

A number of issues exist or will emerge in holistic nursing's future. Acceptance of holistic nursing's legitimacy, both within nursing as well as other disciplines, is one of the most pressing issues today. Other issues can be categorized into education, research, clinical practice, and policy. It is important to note that because many of these issues face not only holistic nursing but other disciplines as well, an interdisciplinary approach is imperative for success in achieving the desired outcomes.

The content in this appendix is not current and is of historical significance only.

Education

There are several areas of educational challenge in the holistic arena. With increased use of complementary and alternative therapies by the American public, both students and faculty need knowledge and skill in their use. Of priority is the integration of holistic relationship-centered philosophies and complementary and alternative modalities into nursing curricula. Core content appropriate for both basic and advanced practice programs needs to be identified, and models for integration of both content and practice experiences into existing curricula are necessary. An elective course is not sufficient to imbue this knowledge to future practitioners of nursing. Holistic nurses will need to work with the accrediting bodies of degree programs to ensure that this content is included in educational programs. There is a definitive need for increased scholarship and financial aid to support training in this area. Faculty development programs also will be necessary to support faculty in understanding and integrating holistic philosophy and practices throughout the curriculum.

Licensure and credentialing provide another challenge for holistic nursing. As complementary/alternative medicine has gained national recognition, state boards of nursing began to attend to the regulation issues. In 2001, Captain Andrew Sparber of the U.S. Public Health Service conducted a study to ascertain the number of boards of nursing that had a formal policy, position, or inclusion of complementary therapies under the scope of practice (Sparber 2001). He found that 25 states (47%) had statements or positions that included specific complementary therapies or examples of these practices, 7 (13%) were discussing the topic, and 21 (40%) had not formally addressed the topic but did not discourage these practices. It will be important in the future to monitor state boards of nursing for evidence of their recognition and support of integrative nursing practice and requirements that include CAM for nursing educational program approval. Finally, holistic nursing has the challenge of working with the state boards to incorporate this content into the National Council Licensure Examination, thus ensuring the credibility of this practice knowledge.

To improve the competency of practitioners and the quality of services, CAM education and training needs to continue beyond basic and advanced academic education. Continuing education programs at national and regional specialty organizations' meetings and conferences

The content in this appendix is not current and is of historical significance only.

may assist in meeting this need. Working with practitioners in other areas of nursing to increase their understanding of the philosophical and theoretical foundations of holistic nursing practices (e.g., intention, presence, and centering) will also be a role of holistic nurses.

Research

Research in the area of holistic nursing will become increasingly important in the future. There is a great need for an evidence base establishing the effectiveness and efficacy of complementary/alternative therapies. However, one of the formidable tasks for nurses will be to identify and describe outcomes of CAM therapies such as healing, well-being, and harmony in order to develop instruments to measure these outcomes. Presently, most outcome measures are based on physical or disease symptomatology. In addition, methodologies need to be expanded to capture the wholeness of the individual's experience, because the philosophy of the CAM therapies rests on a paradigm of wholeness.

Nurses need to address how to secure funding for their holistic research. They need to apply to National Institutes of Health (NIH) centers and Institutes other than just the National Institute of Nursing Research for funding, particularly the National Center for Complementary and Alternative Medicine. But hand in hand with this is the need for nurses to be represented on study sections and review panels to educate and convince the biomedical/NIH community about the value of nursing research; the need for models of research focusing on health promotion and disease prevention, wellness, and self-care instead of just the disease model; and the importance of a variety of designs and research methodologies including qualitative studies, rather than sole reliance on randomized controlled trials.

An area of responsibility for advanced practice holistic nurses is the dissemination of their research findings to various media sources (e.g., television, newsprint) and at non-nursing, interdisciplinary conferences. Publishing in non-nursing journals and serving on editorial boards of non-nursing journals also broadens the appreciation of other disciplines for nursing's role in setting the agenda and conducting research in the area of holism and CAM.

Clinical Practice

Clinical care models reflecting holistic assessment, treatment, health, healing, and caring are important in the development of holistic prac-

The content in this appendix is not current and is of historical significance only.

tice and CAM integration. Implementing holistic and humanistic models in today's healthcare environment will require a paradigm shift for the many providers who subscribe to a disease model of care. Such an acceptance poses an enormous challenge. Holistic nurses with their education and experience are the logical leaders in integrative care and must advance that position.

Addressing the nursing shortage in this country is crucial to the health of our nation. Nurses often leave the profession or frequently change jobs because of unhumanistic and chaotic work environments and professional and personal burnout. Holistic nurses, through their knowledge of caring cultures and stress management techniques, have an extraordinary opportunity to influence and improve the healthcare environments, both for healthcare providers and clients/patients.

Policy

Three major policy issues face holistic nursing in the future: reimbursement, regulation, and access. Public or private policies regarding coverage of and reimbursement for healthcare services play a crucial role in shaping the healthcare system and will play a crucial role in deciding the future of wellness, health promotion, and CAM in the nation's healthcare system. Often CAM is offered as a supplemental benefit rather than as a core or basic benefit, and many third-party payers do not cover such services at all. Coverage of and reimbursement for most services depend on the provider's ability to legally furnish services within the scope of practice. The legal authority to practice is given by the state in which services are provided.

Reimbursement of advanced practice nurses also depends on appropriate credentialing. Holistic nurses will need to work with Medicare and other third-party payers, insurance groups, boards of nursing, healthcare policy makers, legislators, and other professional nursing organizations to ensure that holistic nurses are appropriately reimbursed for services rendered. Another issue regarding reimbursement is the fact that the effectiveness of CAM is influenced by the holistic focus and integrative skill of the provider. Consequently, reimbursement must be included for the process of holistic/integrative care, not just for providing a specific modality.

There are many barriers to the use of holistic therapies by the increasing number of users, providing yet another challenge for holistic nurses.

The content in this appendix is not current and is of historical significance only.

Barriers include lack of awareness of the therapies and their benefits, uncertainty about their effectiveness, inability to pay for them, and limited availability of qualified providers. Access is even more difficult for rural populations; uninsured or underinsured populations; special populations, such as racial and ethnic minorities; and vulnerable populations, such as the elderly and the chronically and terminally ill (WHCCAMP 2002). Holistic nurses have a responsibility to educate the public more fully about health promotion and complementary/alternative modalities and qualified practitioners and to assist people to make informed choices among the array of healthcare alternatives and individual providers. Holistic nurses also must actively participate in the political arena as leaders in this movement to ensure quality, an increased focus on wellness, and access and affordability for all.

Holistic nurses, by developing theoretical and empirical knowledge and caring/healing approaches, will advance holistic nursing practice and education and contribute significantly to the formalization and credibility of this work. They will provide the leadership in the profession in research, the development of educational models, and the integration of a more holistic approach in nursing practice and health care.

The content in this appendix is not current and is of historical significance only.

STANDARDS OF HOLISTIC NURSING PRACTICE

Overarching Philosophical Principles of Holistic Nursing

Holistic nurses express, contribute to, and promote an understanding of the following: a philosophy of nursing that values healing as the desired outcome; the human health experience as a complex, dynamic relationship of health, illness, disease, and wellness; the scientific foundations of nursing practice; and nursing as an art. It is based on the following overarching philosophical tenets that are embedded in every standard of practice.

Principles of Holistic Nursing

The following principles underlie holistic nursing:

Person

- There is unity, totality, and connectedness of everyone and everything (body, mind, emotion, spirit, sexuality, age, environment, social/cultural, belief systems, relationships, context).

- Human beings are unique and inherently good.

- People are able to find meaning and purpose in their own life, experiences, and illness.

- All people have an innate power and capacity for self-healing. Health/illness is subjectively described and determined by the view of the individual. Therefore, the person is honored in all phases of his/her healing process regardless of expectations or outcomes.

- People/persons/individuals identify (are) the recipient(s) of holistic nursing services. These can be clients, patients, families, significant others, populations, or communities. They may be ill and within the healthcare delivery system or well, moving toward personal betterment to enhance well-being.

The content in this appendix is not current and is of historical significance only.

Healing/Health

- Health and illness are natural and a part of life, learning, and movement toward change and development.

- Health is seen as balance, integration, harmony, right relationship, and the betterment of well-being, not just the absence of disease. Healing can take place without cure. The focus is on health promotion/disease prevention/health restoration/lifestyle patterns and habits, as well as symptom relief.

- Illness is considered a teacher and an opportunity for self-awareness and growth as part of the life process. Symptoms are respected as messages.

- People as active partners in the healing process are empowered when they take some control of their own lives, health, and well-being, including personal choices and relationships.

- Treatment is a process that considers the root of the problem, not merely treating the obvious signs and symptoms.

Practice

- Practice is a science (critical thinking, reflection, evidence/research/theory as underlying practice) and an art (intuition, creativity, presence, and self/personal knowing as integral to practice).

- The values and ethic of holism, caring, moral insight, dignity, integrity, competence, responsibility, accountability, and legality underlie holistic nursing practice.

- There are various philosophies and paradigms of health, illness, healing, and approaches/models for the delivery of health care, both in the United States and in other cultures, that need to be understood and utilized.

- Older adults represent the predominant population served by nurses.

- Public policy and the healthcare delivery system influence the health and well-being of society and professional nursing.

The content in this appendix is not current and is of historical significance only.

Nursing Roles

- The nurse is part of the healing environment using warmth, compassion, caring, authenticity, respect, trust, and relationship as instruments of healing in and of themselves.

- Using conventional nursing interventions as well as holistic/complementary/alternative/integrative modalities that enhance the body-mind-emotion-spirit-environment connectedness to foster healing, health, wholenesss, and well-being of people.

- Collaborating and partnering with all constituencies in the health process including the person receiving care and family, community, peers, and other disciplines. Using principles and skills of cooperation, alliance, and respect, and honoring the contributions of all.

- Participating in the change process to develop more caring cultures in which to practice and learn.

- Assisting nurses to nurture and heal themselves.

- Participating in activities that contribute to the improvement of communities and the environment and to the betterment of public health.

- Acting as an advocate for the rights of and equitable distribution and access to health care for all persons, especially vulnerable populations.

- Honoring the ecosystem and our relationship with and need to preserve it, as we are all connected.

Self-Care

- The nurse's self-reflection and self-assessment, self-care, healing, and personal development are necessary for service to others and growth/change in one's own well-being and understanding of one's own personal journey.

- The nurse values oneself and one's calling to holistic nursing as a life purpose.

The content in this appendix is not current and is of historical significance only.

Holistic nursing practice is guided by the holistic caring process, whether used with individuals, families, population groups, or communities. This process involves assessment, diagnosis, outcome identification, planning, implementation, and evaluation. It encompasses all significant actions taken in providing culturally, ethically, respectful, compassionate, and relevant holistic nursing care to all persons.

The content in this appendix is not current and is of historical significance only.

STANDARDS OF PRACTICE

STANDARD 1. ASSESSMENT
The holistic nurse collects comprehensive data pertinent to the person's health or situation.

Measurement Criteria:

The holistic registered nurse:

- Collects comprehensive data including but not limited to physical, functional, psychosocial, emotional, mental, sexual, cultural, age-related, environmental, spiritual/transpersonal, and energy field assessments in a systematic and ongoing process while honoring the uniqueness of the person.

- Identifies areas such as the person's health and cultural practices, values, beliefs, preferences, meanings of health/illness, lifestyle patterns, family issues, and risk behaviors and context.

- Involves the person, family, significant others, caregivers, other healthcare providers, and environment as appropriate in holistic data collection.

- Prioritizes data collection activities based on the person's immediate condition or anticipated needs of the person or situation.

- Uses appropriate evidence-based assessment techniques and instruments in collecting pertinent data as a basis for holistic care.

- Uses analytical models and problem-solving tools.

- Synthesizes available data, information, and knowledge relevant to the situation to identify patterns and variances as they relate to the whole person within the life context.

- Documents and stores relevant data in a retrievable format that is secure and confidential.

- Incorporates various types of knowing, including intuition, when gathering data from the person and validates this intuitive knowledge with the person when appropriate.

Continued ▶

Additional Measurement Criteria for the Holistic Advanced Practice Registered Nurse:

The holistic advanced practice registered nurse:

- Initiates and interprets diagnostic procedures relevant to the person's current status.

- Recognizes the person as the authority on his/her own health experience.

- Elicits and uses client narratives to reveal the context and complexity of the health experience.

- Explores the meanings of the symbolic language expressing itself in areas such as dreams, images, symbols, sensations, and prayers that are a part of the individual's health experience.

STANDARD 2. DIAGNOSIS OR HEALTH ISSUES

The holistic nurse analyzes the assessment data to determine the diagnosis or health issues expressed as actual or potential patterns/problems/needs that are related to health, wellness, disease, or illness.

Measurement Criteria:

The holistic registered nurse:

- Derives the diagnosis or health issues based on holistic assessment data.

- Assists the person to explore the meaning of the health/disease experience.

- Validates the diagnosis or health issues with the person, family/significant other, and other healthcare providers when possible and appropriate.

- Documents diagnoses or health issues in a manner that facilitates the determination of the expected outcomes and plan.

Additional Measurement Criteria for the Holistic Advanced Practice Registered Nurse:

The holistic advanced practice registered nurse:

- Systematically compares and contrasts clinical findings with normal and abnormal variations and development events in formulating a differential diagnosis.

- Utilizes complex data and information obtained during interview, examination, and diagnostic procedures in determining diagnosis.

- Establishes the diagnoses reflecting the level of acuity, severity, and complexity of health patterns/challenges/needs.

- Assists staff in developing and maintaining competency in the diagnostic process.

The content in this appendix is not current and is of historical significance only.

STANDARD 3: OUTCOMES IDENTIFICATION
The holistic registered nurse identifies outcomes for a plan individualized to the person or the situation.

The holistic nurse values the evolution and the process of healing as it unfolds. This implies that specific unfolding outcomes may not be evident immediately due to the non-linear nature of the healing process so that both expected/anticipated and evolving outcomes are considered.

Measurement Criteria:

The holistic registered nurse:

- Involves the person, family, significant others, and other healthcare providers in formulating outcomes when possible and appropriate.

- Derives culturally appropriate outcomes from the diagnoses.

- Considers associated risks, benefits, costs, current scientific evidence, and clinical expertise when formulating outcomes.

- Defines outcomes in terms of the person; the individual's values and beliefs, preferences, age, spiritual practices; ethical considerations, environment, or situation, considering associated risks, benefits, costs, and current scientific evidence.

- Partners with the person to identify realistic goals based on the person's present and potential capabilities and quality of life.

- Assists the person to understand the potential for unfolding outcomes due to the nature of healing.

- Includes a realistic time estimate for attainment of outcomes.

- Develops outcomes that provide direction for continuity of care.

- Modifies outcomes based on changes in the status or preference of the person or evaluation of the situation.

- Documents outcomes as measurable goals.

- Focuses on the person's attaining, maintaining, or regaining health, healing, well-being, or peaceful dying while honoring all phases of her/his healing process regardless of expectations or outcomes.

Additional Measurement Criteria for the Holistic Advanced Practice Registered Nurse:

The holistic advanced practice registered nurse:

- Identifies outcomes that incorporate scientific evidence and are achievable through implementation of evidence-based practices.

- Identifies outcomes that incorporate patient satisfaction, the person's understanding and meanings in their unique patterns and processes, quality of life, cost and clinical effectiveness, and continuity and consistency among providers.

- Supports the use of clinical guidelines for positive outcomes related to the person's healing.

The content in this appendix is not current and is of historical significance only.

STANDARD 4. PLANNING
The holistic registered nurse develops a plan that identifies strategies and alternatives to attain outcomes.

Measurement Criteria:

The holistic registered nurse:

- Develops in partnership with the person an individualized plan considering the person's characteristics or situation including, but not limited to, values, beliefs, spiritual and health practices, preferences, choices, age and cultural appropriateness, environmental sensitivity.

- Develops the plan in conjunction with the person, family, and others, as appropriate.

- Includes strategies within the plan that address each of the identified diagnoses, health issues, or opportunities that may include strategies for promotion and restoration of health and well-being; prevention of illness, injury, and disease; or peaceful dying.

- Collaborates and participates in interdisciplinary/multidisciplinary teams to provide for continuity within the plan.

- Incorporates an implementation pathway or time line within the plan.

- Establishes the plan priorities with the person, family, and others, as appropriate.

- Utilizes the plan to provide direction to other members of the healthcare team.

- Defines the plan to reflect current statutes, rules and regulations, and standards.

- Integrates current trends, research, and evidence-based interventions affecting care in the planning process.

- Considers the economic impact of the plan.

- Includes strategies for health, wholeness, and growth from infant to elder.

The content in this appendix is not current and is of historical significance only.

- Establishes practice settings and safe space and time for both the nurse and person/family/significant others to explore suggested, potential, and alternative options.

- Uses standardized language or recognized terminology to document the plan.

Additional Measurement Criteria for the Holistic Advanced Practice Registered Nurse:

The holistic advanced practice registered nurse:

- Identifies assessment, diagnostic strategies, and therapeutic interventions within the plan and therapeutic effects and side effects that reflect current evidence, including data, research, literature, and expert clinical knowledge and the person's experiences.

- Selects or designs, in partnership with the person, strategies to meet the multifaceted holistic needs of complex individuals.

- Includes the synthesis of the person's values, beliefs, preferences, and choices regarding nursing and medical therapies within the plan.

- Uses linguistic and symbolic language including but not limited to word associations, dreams, storytelling, and journals to explore with individuals the possibilities and options.

The content in this appendix is not current and is of historical significance only.

STANDARD 5. IMPLEMENTATION
The holistic registered nurse implements the identified plan in partnership with the person.

Measurement Criteria:

The holistic registered nurse:

- Partners with the person/family/significant others/caregiver to implement the plan in a safe and timely manner.

- Documents the implementation and any modifications, including changes to or omissions from the identified plan.

- Utilizes evidence-based interventions and treatments specific to the diagnosis or problem.

- Utilizes community resources and systems to implement the plan.

- Collaborates with nursing colleagues and others to implement the plan.

- Promotes the person's capacity for the highest level of participation and problem solving, honoring the person's choices and unique healing journey.

Additional Measurement Criteria for the Holistic Advanced Practice Registered Nurse:

The holistic advanced practice registered nurse:

- Facilitates utilization of systems and community resources to implement the plan.

- Supports collaboration with nursing colleagues and other disciplines to implement the plan for individuals, families, groups, and communities that integrates biomedical, complementary, and alternative approaches to healing.

- Incorporates new knowledge and strategies to initiate change in nursing care practices if desired outcomes are not achieved.

The content in this appendix is not current and is of historical significance only.

STANDARD 5A: COORDINATION OF CARE
The holistic registered nurse coordinates care delivery.

Measurement Criteria:

The holistic registered nurse:

- Coordinates implementation of the plan.

- Documents the coordination of the care.

- Assists the person to recognize alternatives by identifying options for care choices.

Additional Measurement Criteria for the Holistic Advanced Practice Registered Nurse:

The holistic advanced practice registered nurse:

- Provides leadership in the coordination of multidisciplinary health care for integrated delivery of person care services.

- Synthesizes data and information to prescribe necessary system and community support measures, including environmental modifications.

- Coordinates system, environmental, human, and community re-sources that enhance delivery of care across continuums and over time.

STANDARD 5B: HEALTH TEACHING AND HEALTH PROMOTION
The holistic registered nurse employs strategies to promote holistic health/wellness and a safe environment.

Measurement Criteria:

The holistic registered nurse:

- Provides health teaching to individuals, families, and significant others or caregivers that enhances the body-mind-emotion-spirit-environment connection by addressing such topics as:
  - Healthy lifestyles
  - Risk-reducing behaviors
  - Developmental need
  - Activities of daily living
  - Preventive self-care
  - Living with changes secondary to illness and treatment
  - Stress management
  - Opportunities to enhance well-being

- Uses health promotion and health teaching methods appropriate to the situation and the individual's values, beliefs, health practices, age, learning needs, readiness and ability to learn, language preference, spirituality, culture, and socioeconomic status.

- Seeks ongoing opportunities for feedback and evaluation of the effectiveness of the strategies used.

- Educates others by demonstrating a holistic philosophy and ethic that value all ways of knowing and learning.

- Provides appropriate information including but not limited to intended effects and potential adverse effects of the proposed prescribed agents/treatments, costs, complementary/alternative/holistic treatments and procedures, and the effects of single and multiple interventions on the person's health and functioning.

- Assists others to access their own inner wisdom that may provide opportunities to enhance and support growth, development, and wholeness.

The content in this appendix is not current and is of historical significance only.

Additional Measurement Criteria for the Holistic Advanced Practice Registered Nurse:

The holistic advanced practice registered nurse:

- Synthesizes empirical evidence on risk behaviors, decision-making about life choices, learning theories, behavioral change theories, motivational theories, epidemiology, and other related theories and frameworks when designing holistic health information and education.

- Designs health information and education appropriate to the individual's developmental level, learning needs, readiness to learn, and cultural values and beliefs.

- Evaluates health information resources, such as the Internet, within the area of practice for accuracy, readability, and comprehensibility to help the person access quality health information.

- Creates educational environments that are safe for the exploration necessary for learning.

The content in this appendix is not current and is of historical significance only.

STANDARD 5C: CONSULTATION

The holistic advanced practice registered nurse provides consultation to influence the identified plan, enhance the abilities of others, and effect change.

Measurement Criteria for the Holistic Advanced Practice Registered Nurse:

The holistic advanced practice registered nurse:

- Synthesizes clinical data, theoretical frameworks, organizational structures, belief/value systems, and evidence when providing consultation.

- Facilitates the effectiveness of a consultation by involving all stakeholders including the individual in decision-making and negotiating role responsibilities.

- Communicates consultation recommendations that facilitate change.

The content in this appendix is not current and is of historical significance only.

STANDARD 5D: PRESCRIPTIVE AUTHORITY AND TREATMENT

The holistic advanced practice registered nurse uses prescriptive authority, procedures, referrals, treatments, and therapies in accordance with state and federal laws and regulations.

Measurement Criteria for the Holistic Advanced Practice Registered Nurse:

The holistic advanced practice registered nurse:

- Prescribes treatments, therapies, and procedures based on evidence, research, current knowledge, and practice considering the person's holistic healthcare needs and choices.

- Prescribes pharmacologic agents based on a current knowledge of pharmacology and physiology.

- Uses advanced knowledge of pharmacology, psychoneuro-immunology, nutritional supplements, herbal and homeopathic remedies, and a variety of complementary and alternative therapies in prescribing.

- Prescribes specific pharmacologic agents and/or treatments based on: clinical indicators; the person's status, needs, and age; the results of diagnostic and laboratory tests; and the person's beliefs, values, and choices.

- Prescribes holistic therapies that enhance body-mind-emotion-spirit-environment connectedness and foster healing and wholeness.

- Evaluates therapeutic and potential adverse effects of pharmacological and non-pharmacological treatments including but not limited to drug/herbal/homeopathic regimens as well as drug/herbal/homeopathic side effects and interactions.

- Provides individuals with information about intended effects and potential adverse effects of proposed prescriptive therapies.

- Analyzes the effects of single and multiple interventions on the person's health and functioning.

- Provides information about costs and alternative treatments and procedures, as appropriate.

The content in this appendix is not current and is of historical significance only.

STANDARD 6: EVALUATION

The holistic registered nurse evaluates progress toward attainment of outcomes while recognizing and honoring the continuing holistic nature of the healing process.

Measurement Criteria:

The holistic registered nurse:

- Conducts a holistic, systematic, ongoing, and criterion-based evaluation of the outcomes in relation to the structures and processes prescribed by the plan and the indicated time line.

- Collaborates with the person and others involved in the care or situation in the evaluative process.

- Evaluates, in partnership with the person, the effectiveness of the planned strategies in relation to the person's responses and the attainment of the expected and unfolding outcomes.

- Documents the results of the evaluation.

- Uses ongoing assessment data to mutually revise, with the person, family, and health team, the diagnoses, outcomes, plan, and the implementation, as needed.

- Disseminates the results to the person and others involved in the care or situation as appropriate, in accordance with state and federal laws and regulations.

Additional Measurement Criteria for the Holistic Advanced Practice Registered Nurse:

The holistic advanced practice registered nurse:

- Evaluates in partnership with the person the accuracy of the diagnosis and the effectiveness of the interventions in relationship to the person's attainment of expected and evolving outcomes and changes of meaning in the person's health experience.

- Synthesizes the results of the evaluation analyses to determine the impact of the plan on the affected individuals, families, groups, communities, and institutions.

- Uses the results of the evaluation analyses to make or recommend process or structural changes, including policy, procedure, and/or protocol documentation, as appropriate to improve holistic care.

The content in this appendix is not current and is of historical significance only.

Standards of Professional Performance

Standard 7: Quality of Practice
The holistic registered nurse systematically enhances the quality and effectiveness of holistic nursing practice.

Measurement Criteria:

The holistic registered nurse:

- Demonstrates quality by documenting the application of the nursing process in a responsible, accountable, and ethical manner.

- Uses the results of quality improvement activities to initiate changes in holistic nursing practice and in the healthcare delivery system.

- Uses creativity and innovation in holistic nursing practice to improve care delivery.

- Incorporates new knowledge to initiate changes in holistic nursing practice if desired outcomes are not achieved.

- Participates in quality improvement activities for holistic nursing practice. Such activities may include:

  - Identifying aspects of practice important for quality monitoring

  - Using indicators developed to monitor quality and effectiveness of holistic nursing practice

  - Collecting data to monitor quality and effectiveness of holistic nursing practice

  - Analyzing quality data to identify opportunities for improving holistic nursing practice

  - Formulating recommendations to improve holistic nursing practice or outcomes

  - Implementing activities to enhance the quality of holistic nursing practice

  - Developing, implementing, and evaluating policies, procedures, and/or guidelines to improve the quality of practice

Continued ▶

The content in this appendix is not current and is of historical significance only.

- Participating on interdisciplinary teams to evaluate clinical care or health services

- Participating in efforts to minimize costs and unnecessary duplication

- Analyzing factors related to safety, satisfaction, effectiveness, and cost/benefit options

- Analyzing organizational systems for barriers

- Implementing processes to remove or decrease barriers to holistic care within organizational systems

- Working toward creating organizations that value sacred space and environments that enhance healing

Additional Measurement Criteria for the Holistic Advanced Practice Registered Nurse:

The holistic advanced practice registered nurse:

- Obtains and maintains professional certification in the area of expertise.

- Develops indicators to monitor quality and effectiveness of holistic nursing practice.

- Designs quality improvement initiatives.

- Implements initiatives to evaluate the need for change.

- Evaluates the practice environment and quality of holistic nursing care rendered in relation to existing evidence and feedback from individuals and significant others, identifying opportunities for the generation and use of research.

The content in this appendix is not current and is of historical significance only.

STANDARD 8: EDUCATION
The holistic registered nurse attains knowledge and competency that reflects current nursing practice.

Measurement Criteria:

The holistic registered nurse:

- Participates in ongoing educational activities related to appropriate knowledge bases for holistic care and professional issues.

- Demonstrates a commitment to lifelong learning through self-reflection and inquiry to identify learning and personal growth needs.

- Seeks experiences that reflect current practice and population/age-related needs in order to maintain skills and competence in clinical practice and dimensions of the holistic nurse role.

- Acquires knowledge and skills appropriate to the holistic nursing specialty area, practice setting, role, or situation.

- Maintains professional records that provide evidence of competency and lifelong learning.

- Seeks experiences and formal and independent learning activities to maintain and develop clinical and professional skills and knowledge and personal growth.

Additional Measurement Criteria for the Holistic Advanced Practice Registered Nurse:

The holistic advanced practice registered nurse:

- Uses current healthcare research findings and other evidence to expand clinical knowledge, enhance role performance, and increase knowledge of professional issues and changes in national standards for practice and trends in holistic care.

The content in this appendix is not current and is of historical significance only.

Standard 9: Professional Practice Evaluation

The holistic registered nurse evaluates one's own nursing practice in relation to professional practice standards and guidelines, relevant statutes, rules, and regulations.

Measurement Criteria:

The holistic registered nurse's practice reflects the application of knowledge of current practice standards, guidelines, statutes, rules, and regulations.

The holistic registered nurse:

- Reflects on one's practice and how one's own personal, cultural, and/or spiritual beliefs, experiences, biases, education, and values may affect care given to individuals/families/communities.

- Provides age-appropriate care from infant to elder in a culturally and ethnically sensitive manner.

- Engages in self-evaluation of practice on a regular basis, identifying areas of strength as well as areas in which professional development and personal growth would be beneficial.

- Obtains informal feedback regarding one's own holistic practice from individuals receiving care, peers, professional colleagues, and others.

- Participates in systematic peer review as appropriate.

- Takes action to achieve goals identified from evaluation process.

- Provides rationales for practice beliefs, decisions, and actions as part of the informal and formal evaluation processes.

Additional Measurement Criteria for the Holistic Advanced Practice Registered Nurse:

The holistic advanced practice registered nurse:

- Engages in a formal process, seeking feedback regarding one's own practice from individuals receiving care, peers, professional colleagues, and others.

The content in this appendix is not current and is of historical significance only.

STANDARD 10: COLLEGIALITY
The holistic registered nurse interacts with and contributes to the professional development of peers and colleagues.

Measurement Criteria:

The holistic registered nurse:

- Shares knowledge and skills with peers and colleagues as evidenced by such activities as patient care conferences or presentations at formal or informal meetings.

- Recognizes expertise and competency of diverse disciplines and approaches to health care.

- Provides peers with feedback regarding their practice and/or role performance in a constructive and sincere manner.

- Interacts with peers and colleagues to enhance one's own holistic nursing practice, personal development, and/or role performance.

- Maintains compassionate and caring relationships with peers and colleagues.

- Contributes to an environment that is conducive to enhancing the education of healthcare professionals about holism.

- Promotes work environments conducive to support, understanding, respect, health, healing, caring, wholeness, and harmony.

Additional Measurement Criteria for the Holistic Advanced Practice Registered Nurse:

The holistic advanced practice registered nurse:

- Models expert holistic nursing practice to interdisciplinary team members and healthcare consumers.

- Mentors other registered nurses and colleagues as appropriate.

- Participates with interdisciplinary teams that contribute to role development and advanced holistic nursing practice and holistic health care.

- Establishes practice environments that recognize and value holistic communication as fundamental to holistic care.

The content in this appendix is not current and is of historical significance only.

STANDARD 11: COLLABORATION
The holistic registered nurse collaborates with the person, family, and others in the conduct of holistic nursing practice.

Measurement Criteria:

The holistic registered nurse:

- Communicates with the person, family, significant others, caregivers, and interdisciplinary healthcare providers regarding the person's care and the holistic nurse's role in the provision of that care.

- Collaborates in creating a documented plan, focused on outcomes and decisions related to care and delivery of services, that indicates communication with individuals receiving care, families, and others as appropriate.

- Partners with others to enhance holistic care in order to effect change and generate positive outcomes through knowledge of the person or situation.

- Documents referrals, including provisions for continuity of care.

- Understands, utilizes, and refers to a range of approaches and therapies from diverse disciplines and systems of care as appropriate.

Additional Measurement Criteria for the Holistic Advanced Practice Registered Nurse:

The holistic advanced practice registered nurse:

- Partners with other disciplines to enhance holistic care through interdisciplinary activities such as education, consultation, management, technological development, or research opportunities.

- Facilitates an interdisciplinary process with other members of the healthcare team that enhances the contribution of all.

- Documents plan, communications, rationales for plan changes, and collaborative discussions.

- Facilitates the negotiation of holistic/complementary/alternative/ integrative and conventional healthcare services for continuity of care and program planning.

The content in this appendix is not current and is of historical significance only.

STANDARD 12: ETHICS
The holistic registered nurse integrates ethical provisions in all areas of practice.

Measurement Criteria:

The holistic registered nurse:

- Uses *Code of Ethics for Nurses with Interpretive Statements* (ANA 2001) and *Position Statement on Holistic Nursing Ethics* (AHNA 2007) to guide practice and articulate the moral foundation of holistic nursing.

- Identifies the ethics of caring and its contribution to unity of self, others, nature, and God/Life Force/Absolute/Transcendent as central to holistic nursing practice.

- Delivers care in a manner that preserves and protects the person's autonomy, dignity, rights, values, and beliefs.

- Protects and maintains the person's personal privacy and confidentiality within legal and regulatory parameters.

- Respects the person's choices and health trajectory, which may be incongruent with conventional wisdom.

- Serves as an advocate in assisting the person in developing skills for self-advocacy and making educated choices about his/her care.

- Maintains a therapeutic and professional person–nurse relationship with appropriate professional role boundaries.

- Engages in self-assessment and demonstrates a commitment to practicing self-care strategies to enhance physical, psychological, intellectual, sociological, and spiritual well-being, manage stress, and connect with self and others.

- Contributes to resolving ethical issues of individuals, colleagues, or systems as evidenced in such activities as participating on ethics committees.

- Reports illegal, incompetent, or impaired practices.

- Recognizes that the well-being of the ecosystem of the planet is a determining condition for the well-being of human beings.

Continued ▶

- Engages in activities that respect, nurture, and enhance the integral relationship with the earth, and advocates for the well-being of the global community's economy, education, and social justice.

- Advocates for the rights of vulnerable, repressed, or underserved populations by such activities as:

  - Acting on behalf of individuals, families, groups, and communities who cannot seek or demand ethical treatment on their own

  - Seeking to eliminate barriers such as affordability and accessibility that create added risks for persons of varied racial, ethnic, and social backgrounds, as well as the elderly and children

  - Advocating for other nurses and colleagues

- Values all life experiences as opportunities to find personal meaning and cultivate self-awareness, self-reflection, and growth.

Additional Measurement Criteria for the Holistic Advanced Practice Registered Nurse:

The holistic advanced practice registered nurse:

- Informs the person of the risks, benefits, and outcomes of health-care regimens.

- Participates in interdisciplinary teams that address ethical risks, benefits, and outcomes.

- Engages others to incorporate a holistic perspective of ethical situations and decision-making.

- Actively contributes to creating an ecosystem that supports well-being for all life.

STANDARD 13: RESEARCH
The holistic registered nurse integrates research into practice.

Measurement Criteria:

The holistic registered nurse:

- Utilizes the best available evidence, including theories and research findings, to guide practice decisions.

- Actively and ethically participates in research activities related to holistic health at various levels appropriate to the holistic nurse's level of education and position. Such activities may include:

  - Identifying problems specific to nursing research (person care and nursing practice)

  - Participating in data collection (surveys, pilot projects, formal studies)

  - Participating in a formal committee or program

  - Sharing research activities and/or findings with individuals/families/peers, those in other disciplines, and others

  - Systematically inquiring into healing, wholeness, cultural, spiritual, and health issues by conducting research or supporting and utilizing the research of others

  - Critically analyzing and interpreting research for application to holistic practice

  - Using research findings in the development of policies, procedures, and standards of practice in holistic person care

  - Incorporating research as a basis for learning

- Contributes to conducting research and applying research findings that link environmental hazards and human response patterns.

Continued ▶

The content in this appendix is not current and is of historical significance only.

Additional Measurement Criteria for the Holistic Advanced Practice Registered Nurse:

The holistic advanced practice registered nurse:

- Contributes to nursing knowledge by conducting or synthesizing research that discovers, examines, and evaluates knowledge, theories, philosophies, context, criteria, and creative approaches to improve holistic healthcare practice.

- Formally disseminates research findings through activities such as presentations, publications, consultations, and journal clubs for a variety of audiences including nursing, other disciplines, and the public to improve holistic care and further develop the foundation and practice of holistic nursing.

- Creates ways to study the integration of body-mind-emotion-spirit-environment therapies to achieve optimal care outcomes.

- Participates with others to identify research questions or areas for inquiry and set research priorities that have high significance in understanding and/or improving health/wellness promotion and disease prevention; the quality of life; spirituality; cultural beliefs and health practices; and healing and well-being.

The content in this appendix is not current and is of historical significance only.

STANDARD 14: RESOURCE UTILIZATION

The holistic registered nurse considers factors related to safety, effectiveness, cost, and impact on practice in the planning and delivery of nursing services.

Measurement Criteria:

The holistic registered nurse:

- Evaluates factors such as safety, effectiveness, availability, cost and benefits, efficiencies, and impact on practice when choosing practice options that would result in the same expected outcome.

- Assists the person, family, and significant others or caregivers, as appropriate, in identifying and securing appropriate and available services to address health-related needs.

- Identifies discriminatory healthcare practices as they impact the person and engages in effective nondiscriminatory practices.

- Assigns or delegates tasks based on the needs and condition of the person, potential for harm, stability of the person's condition, complexity of the task, and predictability of the outcome.

- Assists the person, family, and significant others in becoming informed consumers about the health promotion options, costs, risks, and benefits of treatment and care.

Additional Measurement Criteria for the Holistic Advanced Practice Registered Nurse:

The holistic advanced practice registered nurse:

- Utilizes organizational and community resources to formulate multidisciplinary or interdisciplinary plans of care.

- Develops innovative solutions for the person's care needs/challenges/problems that address effective resource utilization and maintenance of quality.

- Develops evaluation strategies to demonstrate cost effectiveness, cost benefit, and efficiency factors associated with holistic nursing practice.

The content in this appendix is not current and is of historical significance only.

STANDARD 15: LEADERSHIP

The holistic registered nurse provides leadership in the professional practice setting and the profession.

Measurement Criteria:

The holistic registered nurse:

- Engages in teamwork as a team player and a team builder.

- Works to create and maintain healthy work environments conducive to enhancing healing, wholeness, and harmony in local, regional, national, or international communities.

- Displays the ability to define a clear vision, associated goals, and a plan to implement and measure progress toward holistic health care.

- Demonstrates a commitment to continuous, lifelong learning and personal growth for self and others.

- Teaches others to succeed, by mentoring and other strategies.

- Exhibits creativity and flexibility through times of change.

- Demonstrates energy, excitement, and a passion for quality holistic work.

- Willingly accepts mistakes by self and others, thereby creating a culture in which risk-taking is both safe and expected.

- Inspires loyalty through valuing of people as the most precious asset in an organization.

- Directs the coordination of care across settings and among caregivers, including oversight of licensed and unlicensed personnel in any assigned or delegated tasks.

- Serves in key roles in the work setting to advance the philosophy and role of holistic nursing by participating on committees, councils, and administrative teams.

- Promotes advancement of the profession through participation in professional organizations and focusing on strategies that bring unity and healing to the nursing profession.

- Engages in local, state, national, and international levels to expand the knowledge and practice of holistic nursing and awareness of holistic health issues.

The content in this appendix is not current and is of historical significance only.

Additional Measurement Criteria for the Holistic Advanced Practice Registered Nurse:

The holistic advanced practice registered nurse:

- Works to influence decision-making bodies to improve holistic, integrated care.

- Provides direction to enhance the effectiveness of the healthcare team.

- Initiates and revises protocols or guidelines to reflect evidence-based practice, to reflect accepted changes in care management, or to address emerging problems such as the growing elderly population.

- Promotes communication of information and advancement of the profession and holistic nursing through writing, publishing, and presentations for professional or lay/public audiences.

- Designs innovations to effect change in practice and to improve holistic health outcomes.

- Articulates the ideas underpinning holistic nursing philosophy, placing these ideas in a historical, philosophical, and scientific context while projecting future trends in thinking by such activities as:

  - Applying, teaching, mentoring, and leading others in developing holistic care models and providing holistic integrated care

  - Leading organizations in creating therapeutic environments that value holistic caring, social support, and healing, where individuals feel connected, supported, and valued

  - Understanding the political, social, organizational, and financial barriers to holistic care for individuals, population groups, and communities and working to eliminate these barriers while balancing justice with compassion

  - Sharing knowledge and understanding of a wide range of cultural norms and healthcare practices/beliefs/values concerning individuals, families, groups, and communities from varied racial, ethnic, spiritual, and social backgrounds

Continued ▶

- Acting as a leader, collaborator, consultant, and change agent in evaluating global health issues and environmental safety, anticipating the potential effect of environmental hazards on the health or welfare of individuals, groups, and communities, and assisting in reducing or eliminating environmental hazards

The content in this appendix is not current and is of historical significance only.

REFERENCES

American Association of Colleges of Nursing. (1996). *The essentials of master's education for advanced practice nursing.* Washington, DC: AACN.

American Holistic Nurses Association. (1998). *Description of holistic nursing.* Flagstaff, AZ: AHNA.

American Holistic Nurses Association. (2005). *Standards of holistic nursing practice.* Flagstaff, AZ: AHNA.

American Holistic Nurses Association. (2005). *Standards of advanced holistic nursing practice for graduate-prepared nurses.* Flagstaff, AZ: AHNA.

American Holistic Nurses Association. (2007). *Position statement on holistic nursing ethics.* Flagstaff, AZ: AHNA.

American Nurses Association. (1996). *Scope and standards of advanced practice registered nursing practice.* Washington, DC: American Nurses Publishing.

American Nurses Association. (2001). *Code of ethics for nurses with interpretive statements.* Washington, DC: American Nurses Publishing.

American Nurses Association. (2003). *Nursing's social policy statement,* 2nd ed. Silver Spring, MD: Nursesbooks.org.

American Nurses Association. (2004). *Nursing: Scope and standards of practice.* Silver Spring, MD: Nursesbooks.org.

Barnes, P.M., E. Powell-Griner, K. McFann, & R.L. Nahin. (2004). Complementary and alternative medicine use among adults: United States, 2002. *Advance data from vital and health statistics,* No. 243, May 27, 2004. Hyattsville, MD: U.S. Department of Health and Human Services, Centers for Disease Control and Prevention, and National Center for

The content in this appendix is not current and is of historical significance only.

Alternative and Complementary Medicine. (Available online: http://www.mbcrc.med.ucla.edu/PDFs/camsurvey2.pdf)

Dossey, B., L. Keagan, & C. Guzzetta. (2005). *Holistic nursing: A handbook for practice,* 4th ed. Sudbury, MA: Jones and Bartlett.

Eisenberg, D.M., R. C. Kessler, C. Foster, F. E. Norlock, D.R. Calkins, & T.L. Delbanco. (1993). Unconventional medicine in the United States: Prevalence, costs, and patterns of use. *New England Journal of Medicine* 328(4): 246–252. (Abstract and citations available online: http://content.nejm.org/cgi/content/short/328/4/246)

Eisenberg, D., R. B. Davis, S.L. Ettner, S. Appel, S. Wiilke, M. Van Rompay, & R. C. Kessler. (1998). Trends in alternative medicine use in the United States, 1990–1997. *Journal of the American Medical Association* 280: 1569–75.

Eliopoulos, C. (2005). *Nurse competency in aging: Safe integration of complementary and alternative therapies in geriatric care.* Flagstaff, AZ: American Holistic Nurses Association.

Fenton, M., and D. Morris. (2003). The integration of holistic nursing practices and complementary and alternative modalities into curricula of schools of nursing. *Alternative Therapies in Health and Nursing* 9(4): 62–67.

Frisch, N., B. Dossey, C. Guzzetta, and J. Quinn. (2000). *Standards of holistic nursing practice with guidelines for caring and healing.* Gaithersburg, MD: Aspen.

Guzzetta, C., ed. (1998). *Essential readings in holistic nursing.* Gaithersburg, MD: Aspen.

Health Forum. (2006). *Report of hospitals using complementary and alternative medicine.* Chicago: American Hospital Association.

Institute of Medicine. (2005). *Complementary and alternative medicine in the United States.* Washington, DC: The National Academies Press.

The content in this appendix is not current and is of historical significance only.

Mariano, C. (2003). Advanced practice in holistic nursing, in *Nurse practitioners: Evolution of advanced practice,* 4th ed., ed. M. Mezey, D. McGivern, & E. Sullivan-Marx, pp. 233–253. New York : Springer Publishing Company.

National Center for Complementary and Alternative Medicine. (2005). *Expanding horizons of health care: Strategic plan 2005–2009.* Washington, DC: National Institutes of Health.

National Institutes of Health. (2000). *Expanding horizons of health care (2001–2005): National Center for Complementary and Alternative Medicine's Five-Year Strategic Plan.* Bethesda, MD: NIH.

Shelky, M. (2005). *Nurse competency in aging. Aging with chronicity: Overview and resources.* Flagstaff, AZ: American Holistic Nurses Association.

Sparber, A. (2001). State boards of nursing and scope of practice of registered nurses performing complementary therapies. *Online Journal of Issues in Nursing,* 6(3), Manuscript 10. Retrieved from http://www.nursingworld.org/ojin/topic15/tpc15_6.htm

Tresolini, C.P., & Pew-Fetzer Task Force. (1994). *Health professions education and relationship-centered care: Report of the Pew-Fetzer Task Force on advancing psychosocial health education.* San Francisco, CA: Pew Health Professions Commission. (Available online at http://www.futurehealth.ucsf.edu/pdf_files/RelationshipCentered.pdf)

U.S. Department of Health and Human Services. (1999a). *The patients' bill of rights in Medicare and Medicaid.* Accessed on January 1, 2007, at http://www.hhs.gov/news/press/1999pres/990412.html

U.S. Department of Health and Human Services. (1999b). *National health interview survey 1999.* Centers for Disease Control and Prevention. National Center for Health Statistics. Division of Health Interview Statistics. Hyattsville. MD: U.S. DHHS.

U.S. Department of Health and Human Services. (2005). *Healthy People 2010: Midcourse review.* U.S. DHHS 2005. Available online at http://www.healthypeople.gov/data/midcourse/default.htm

The content in this appendix is not current and is of historical significance only.

Watson, J. (2005). *Caring science as sacred science.* Philadelphia: F.A. Davis.

Weeks, J. (2001). Foreword, in *Mosby's complementary and alternative medicine: A research-based approach,* eds. L. W. Freeman & G.F. Lawlis. St. Louis: Mosby.

White House Commission on Complementary and Alternative Medicine Policy (WHCCAMP). (2001). Interim progress report. *Alternative Therapies in Health and Medicine* 7(6): 32–40.

White House Commission on Complementary and Alternative Medicine Policy (WHCCAMP). (2002). *Final report.* Washington, DC: U.S. Government Printing Office.

The content in this appendix is not current and is of historical significance only.

BIBLIOGRAPHY

American Holistic Nurses Association. (2005). *Standards of holistic nursing practice*. Flagstaff, AZ: AHNA. (Included as Appendix B in this book starting, on page 81)

American Holistic Nurses Association. (2005). *Standards of advanced holistic nursing practice for graduate prepared nurses*. Flagstaff, AZ: AHNA. (Included as Appendix C in this book, starting on page 93)

American Holistic Nurses Association (2007). *Position on nursing research and scholarship*. Flagstaff, AZ: AHNA.

American Holistic Nurses Association. (2007). *Position on the role of nurses in the practice of complementary and alternative therapies*. Flagstaff, AZ: AHNA.

Dossey, B., ed. (1997). *Core curriculum for holistic nursing*. Gaithersburg, MD: Aspen.

Dossey, B., L. Keagan, and C. Guzzetta. (2005). *Holistic nursing: A handbook for practice,* 4th ed. Gaithersburg, MD: Aspen.

Frisch, N., B. Dossey, C. Guzzetta, and J. Quinn. (2000). AHNA *standards of holistic nursing practice: Guidelines for caring and healing*. Gaithersburg, MD: Aspen.

Guzzetta, C., ed. (1998). *Essential readings in holistic nursing*. Gaithersburg, MD: Aspen.

Mariano, C. (2003). Advanced practice in holistic nursing, in *Nurse practitioners: Evolution of advanced practice,* 4th ed., eds. M. Mezey, D. McGivern, & E. Sullivan-Marx. New York: Springer Publishing Company.

Mariano, C. (2005). An overview of holistic nursing. *Imprint* 52(2): 1148–52.

Watson, J. (2004). *Caring science as sacred science*. Philadelphia: F.A. Davis.

Appendix B.

Goals and Activities of the American Holistic Nurses Association (AHNA)

The goals and endeavors of the AHNA have continued to map conceptual frameworks and the blueprint for holistic nursing practice, education, and research, which is the most complete way to conceptualize and practice professional nursing. Beginning in 1993, AHNA undertook an organization development process that included the following areas:

- Identification of the steps toward national certification in 1993–1994.

- Revision of the 1990 *Standards of Holistic Nursing Practice*, completed in 1995.

- Completing a role delineation study, *Inventory of Professional Activities and Knowledge Statements of a Holistic Nurse* (also known as the IPAKHN Survey) in 1997.

- Developing a national Holistic Nursing Certification Examination, completed in 1997.

- Completing major revisions of the 1995 *Standards of Holistic Nursing Practice* in 1999, with additional editorial changes in January 2000 and 2005.

- Developing a Core Curriculum for basic holistic nursing based on the Basic Standards (1997).

- Approving and adopting *Standards of Advanced Holistic Nursing Practice for Graduate-Prepared Nurses* (2002, revised 2005).

- Developing a Core Curriculum for advanced holistic nursing based on the Advanced Standards (2003).

- Developing the Certification Exam for Advanced Holistic Nursing Practice by The American Holistic Nurses Certification Corporation (AHNCC) in 2004. This exam was first offered in March 2005.

- Revising the 2005 Basic and Advanced *Standards of Holistic Nursing Practice* to meet ANA criteria for recognition of holistic nursing as a specialty.

- Applying for and obtaining recognition of holistic nursing as official specialty within nursing by ANA (2006).

- Publishing *Holistic Nursing: Scope and Standards of Practice* (2007).

- Participating in the revision of the revised AACN *Essentials of Baccalaureate Education for Professional Nursing Practice* to incorporate holistic nursing principles and practices (2008).

- Developing a web site for holistic geriatric care (2009).

- Becoming an affiliate member of ANA (2011).

- Partnering in the national Joining Forces Campaign (2012).

Other AHNA activities that support and promote holistic nursing include:

- Collaborating with other organizations to strengthen the voice of nursing

- Educating the public about integrative therapies and holistic practitioners

- Endorsing certificate programs for nurses that have content in holistic nursing, healing, and/or complementary/alternative/integrative modalities

- Organizing networking groups nationally and internationally to further holistic nursing

- Providing and approving continuing education programs featuring holistic health topics, holistic research, and holistic education

- Integrating holistic content and practices into academic nursing curricula

- Improving the healthcare workplace by promoting the incorporation of the concepts of holistic nursing, self-care, and wellness

- Development of evidence-based holistic/integrative practice through research and dissemination

- Granting awards for holistic nursing research and holistic nursing education

- Awarding student scholarships

- Publishing several informational, educational, research, and professional support materials such as *Beginnings; JHN*; and Research, Membership, Faculty-Student, and Practice e-newsletters

- Monitoring and responding to legislative policy issues

- Advocating for a focus on wellness, health promotion, and access to affordable care

Membership in the AHNA is open to all individuals who support the mission of the organization. AHNA's philosophy is that holistic nursing is the *heart* of nursing and the *science* of holism.

Appendix C.

Categories of Complementary/ Alternative/Integrative/ Modalities (CAM) Therapies

Natural products. This area includes substances found in nature, such as a variety of herbal medicines (also known as *botanicals*), vitamins, minerals, whole diet therapies, and other "natural products." Many are sold over the counter as dietary supplements. (Some uses of dietary supplements—e.g., taking a multivitamin to meet minimum daily nutritional requirements or taking calcium to promote bone health—are not thought of as CAM.) CAM "natural products" also include probiotics—live microorganisms (usually bacteria) that are similar to microorganisms normally found in the human digestive tract and that may have beneficial effects. Probiotics are available in foods (e.g., yogurts) or as dietary supplements.

Mind–body medicine. Mind–body practices focus on the interactions among the brain, mind, body, and behavior, with the intent to use the mind to affect physical functioning and promote health. Many CAM practices embody this concept—in different ways. Some techniques that were considered CAM in the past have become mainstream (for example, patient support groups, psychotherapy, cognitive-behavioral therapy). Mind–body techniques include meditation, relaxation, imagery, hypnotherapy, yoga, biofeedback, and tai chi. Other therapies are autogenic training, spirituality, prayer, mental healing, and therapies that use creative outlets such as art, music, dance, or journaling. Acupuncture is considered to be a part of mind–body medicine, but it is also a component of energy medicine, manipulative and body-based practices, and traditional Chinese medicine.

Manipulative and body-based practices. Manipulative and body-based practices focus primarily on the structures and systems of the body, including the bones and joints, soft tissues, and circulatory and lymphatic systems. Two commonly used therapies fall within this category: spinal manipulation including chiropractic or osteopathic manipulation, and massage.

Movement therapies. CAM also encompasses movement therapies—a broad range of Eastern and Western movement-based approaches used to promote physical, mental, emotional, and spiritual well-being. Examples include Feldenkrais method, Alexander Technique, Pilates, Rolfing Structural Integration, and Trager psychophysical integration.

Practices of traditional healers. Traditional healers use methods based on indigenous theories, beliefs, and experiences handed down from generation to generation. Examples include Native American healer/medicine man, African, Middle Eastern, Tibetan, Central and South American, and Curanderismo.

Energy therapies. Some CAM practices involve manipulation of various energy fields to affect health. Such fields may be characterized as veritable (measurable) or putative (yet to be measured). Practices based on veritable forms of energy include those involving electromagnetic fields (e.g., magnet therapy, light therapy, or alternating-current or direct-current fields). Practices based on putative energy fields (also called *biofields*) generally reflect the concept that human beings are infused with subtle forms of energy. Some forms of energy therapy manipulate biofields by applying pressure, such as acupressure, and manipulating the body by placing the hands in or through these fields. Examples include Gong, Reiki, Therapeutic Touch, and Healing Touch.

Whole medical systems. Complete systems of theory and practice that have evolved over time in different cultures and apart from conventional or Western medicine; may be considered CAM. Examples of ancient whole medical systems include Ayurvedic medicine and traditional Chinese medicine. More modern systems that have developed in the past few centuries include homeopathy and naturopathy.

Source: National Center for Complementary and Alternative Medicine, National Institutes of Health (2011); http://nccam.nih.gov

Appendix D.

AHNA Position Statements

American Holistic Nurses Association. (2012). *Position on Holistic Nursing Ethics*. Flagstaff, AZ: AHNA. www.ahna.org/position statements

American Holistic Nurses Association. (2012). *Position on Nursing Research and Scholarship*. Flagstaff, AZ: AHNA. www.ahna.org/position statements

American Holistic Nurses Association. (2012). *Position on the Role of Nurses in the Practice of Complementary and Alternative Therapies*. Flagstaff, AZ: AHNA. www.ahna.org/position statements

American Holistic Nurses Association. (2009). *White Paper: Research in AHNA*. Flagstaff, AZ: AHNA. www.ahna.org/research white paper

Position on Holistic Nursing Ethics

Code of Ethics for Holistic Nurses

We believe that the fundamental responsibilities of the nurse are to promote health, facilitate healing, and alleviate suffering. The need for nursing is universal. Inherent in nursing is the respect for life, dignity, and the rights of all persons. Nursing care is given a context mindful of the holistic nature of humans, understanding the body-mind-emotion-spirit. Nursing care is unrestricted by considerations of nationality, race, creed, color, age, sex, sexual preference, politics, or social status. Given that nurses practice in culturally diverse settings, professional nurses must have an understanding of the cultural background of clients in order to provide culturally appropriate interventions.

Nurses render services to clients who can be individuals, families, groups, or communities. The client is an active participant in health care and should be included in all nursing care planning decisions.

To provide services to others, each nurse has a responsibility towards the client, co-workers, nursing practice, the profession of nursing, society, and the environment.

Nurses and Self

The nurse has a responsibility to model health care behaviors. Holistic nurses strive to achieve harmony in their own lives and assist others striving to do the same.

Nurses and the Client

The nurse's primary responsibility is to the client needing nursing care. The nurse strives to see the client as whole and provides care that is professionally appropriate and culturally consonant. The nurse holds in confidence all information obtained in professional practice and uses professional judgment in disclosing such information. The nurse enters into a relationship with the client that is guided by mutual respect and a desire for growth and development.

Nurses and Co-Workers

The nurse maintains cooperative relationships with co-workers in nursing and other fields. Nurses have a responsibility to nurture each other and to assist nurses to work as a team in the interest of client care. If a client's care is endangered by a co-worker, the nurse must take appropriate action on behalf of the client.

Nurses and Nursing Practice

The nurse carries personal responsibility for practice and maintaining continued competence. Nurses have the right to use all appropriate nursing interventions and have the obligation to determine the efficacy and safety of all nursing actions. Wherever applicable, nurses use research findings in directing practice.

Nurses and the Profession

The nurse plays a role in determining and implementing desirable standards of nursing practice and education and research. Holistic nurses may assume a leadership position to guide the profession towards a holistic philosophy of practices. Nurses support nursing research and the development of holistically oriented nursing theories. The nurse participates in establishing and maintaining equitable social and economic working conditions in nursing.

Nurses and Society

The nurse, along with other citizens, has the responsibility for initiating and supporting actions to meet the health and social needs of all society.

Nurses and the Environment

Nurses strive to create a client environment to be one of peace, harmony, and nurturance so that healing may take place. The nurse considers the health of the ecosystem in relation to the need for health, safety, and peace of all persons.

Revised and re-approved by AHNA, 2012.

Position on the Role of Nurses in the Practice of Complementary and Alternative Therapies

Overview

Complementary and alternative modalities (CAM) offer therapies that supplement conventional medical care. The National Center on Complementary and Alternative Medicine (NCCAM) of the National Institutes of Health has categorized major domains of CAM practices:

- Natural products such as herbal therapies, diet therapies, nutritional supplements, and vitamins

- Mind–body interventions, such as meditation, relaxation, imagery, hypnosis, yoga, tai chi, prayer, art and music therapies, cognitive-behavioral therapy, biofeedback, therapeutic counseling, and stress management

- Manipulative and body-based methods, such as chiropractic, massage therapy, osteopathy, and reflexology

- Movement therapies such as Feldenkrais method, Alexander Technique, Pilates, Rolfing, dance therapy

- Practices of traditional indigenous healers such as Native American, African, Middle Eastern, Tibetan, and Latin American

- Whole medical systems, such as Ayurveda, traditional Chinese medicine, traditional Oriental medicine, homeopathy, naturopathy

- Energy therapies, such as Therapeutic Touch, Reiki, qi gong, acupressure, Healing Touch, light therapy, and magnet therapy

Holistic care refers to approaches and interventions that address the needs of the whole person: body, mind, emotion, and spirit. Healing arts are those interventions that foster an individual's healing process, i.e., a return of the individual toward a state of wholeness in which body, mind, emotion, and spirit are integrated and balanced, and the person is able to reach deeper levels of personal understanding. Healing does not equate to curing, although they can be synchronous. The nursing profession has a long history of caring for individuals in a holistic manner and integrating the healing arts with conventional treatments. Florence Nightingale recognized the importance of caring for the whole person and encouraged interventions that enhanced individuals' abilities to draw upon their own healing powers. She considered touch, light, aromatics, empathetic listening, music, quiet reflection, and similar healing measures as essential ingredients to good nursing care. Today's education of registered nurses is built upon these same principles.

The American Holistic Nurses Association (AHNA) is a professional nursing association dedicated to the promotion of holism and healing. The AHNA believes that nurses enter therapeutic partnerships with clients, their families, and their communities to serve as facilitators in the healing process. The holistic caring process supported by AHNA is one in which nurses:

- Acquire and maintain current knowledge and competency in holistic nursing practice, including CAM therapies and practices integrated within that practice

- Provide care and guidance to persons through nursing interventions and therapies consistent with research findings and other sound evidence

- Hold to a professional code of ethics and healing that seeks to preserve wholeness and dignity of self and others

- Engage in self-care and further develop their own personal awareness of being an instrument of healing

- Recognize each person as a whole: body-mind-spirit

- Assess clients holistically, using appropriate traditional and holistic methods

- Create a plan of care in collaboration with the clients and their significant others consistent with cultural background, health beliefs, sexual orientation, values, and preferences that focuses on health promotion, recovery or restoration, or peaceful dying so that the person is as independent as possible

Nursing and CAM

The AHNA believes that inherent in the nursing role is the ability to assess, plan, intervene, evaluate, and perform preventive, supportive, and restorative functions of the physical, emotional, mental, and spiritual domains. Therefore, it is expected that the nurse may draw upon and utilize principles and techniques of both conventional and CAM therapies, and that these would be within the scope of nursing practice. AHNA supports the integration of CAM into conventional health care to enable the client to benefit from the best of all treatments available. In their provision of holistic care, nurses employ practices and therapies from both CAM and conventional medicine.

Consistent with conventional nursing practice, nurses must be competent in the CAM therapies and practices they use. The AHNA believes nurses integrate these practices into conventional care as part of a holistic practice. In addition, nurses support and assist clients with their use of CAM provided by other practitioners by:

- Identifying the need for CAM interventions

- Assisting clients in locating providers of CAM interventions

- Facilitating the use of CAM interventions through education, counseling, coaching, and other forms of assistance

- Coordinating the use of CAM among various health care providers involved in clients' care; and evaluating the effectiveness of clients' complete integrative care

AHNA's Position

The AHNA believes that although selected CAM are appropriate interventions for use by nurses, the use of these interventions must be integrated into a comprehensive holistic nursing practice. Practicing within a holistic nursing framework does not imply competency in effectively and safely utilizing CAM therapies and practices. Nurses must be responsible for seeking, when necessary, additional education and experience and demonstrating clinical competency in all interventions used in their nursing practice.

A nurse practicing as a therapist of a specific conventional or CAM therapy must have the education, skills, and credentials ascribed for that therapy. The nurse also must operate within the legal scope of practice of the nurse's licensure and jurisdiction.

AHNA views nurses as being in a unique position in the implementation of CAM throughout the healthcare system in that registered nurses:

- represent the greatest number of healthcare professionals, representing more than 2.7 million healthcare professionals, and are employed in more diverse clinical settings than any other healthcare professional;

- are uniquely prepared to differentiate normality from illness, provide interventions for health promotion and illness-related care, and use a wide range of medical technology and the healing arts;

- are advocates for clients rather than specific products or practices, and therefore are in an excellent position to assure appropriate and adequate use of all types of services; and

- are trusted and held in high esteem by consumers.

These factors support nurses holding a leadership role in the implementation of CAM in various service settings and the coordination of CAM utilization by clients as part of an integrated approach to care.

Revised and re-approved by AHNA, 2012.

Position on Nursing Research and Scholarship

Holistic care refers to approaches and interventions that address the needs of the whole person—body, mind, emotion, and spirit—focusing on healing the whole person as its goal. Nursing is the care and treatment of the human response to actual or potential health problems, concerns, or life processes. Thus, nursing research and scholarship should assist its practitioners to: (1) understand the holistic nature of human experiences of health, healing, and illness; and (2) evaluate the effects of holistic nursing actions on the client's health, healing, illness, and recovery.

Research supporting holistic nursing includes descriptive, explanatory, and exploratory designs that expand our understanding of holistic practice and enhances the evidence base for practice.

Holistic nursing research may be conducted using qualitative, quantitative, mixed methods, or other approaches that further our understanding of phenomena such as the complexity of the human condition, healing, and outcomes of holistic therapies. Research, however, needs to be planned and results interpreted in a holistic, integral, or unitary framework for it to be considered "holistic" nursing research.

Several ways of knowing—rational/scientific, intuitive, and aesthetic—are recognized in holistic nursing research. Nursing scholarship involves intuitive and aesthetic approaches to comprehend the multidimensional nature of our work which encompasses: (1) the art of care, (2) the wholeness of the client's experiences and meaning of patterns that emerge, (3) the beauty of authentic interaction; and (4) the knowledge of that which is perceived through non-verbal, non-objective expression. Nursing scholarship involves rational/empirical understanding that is necessary to demonstrate: (1) basic mechanisms of nursing actions and integrative therapies; (2) clinical safety, efficacy, and treatment outcomes of holistic modalities; and (3) the interactive and integrative nature of body/mind/emotion/spirit.

Many phenomena of concern to nursing remain unknown or undocumented, such that exploratory, qualitative research is a highly effective method for expanding the disciplines' developing body of knowledge. Further, many aspects of the human responses to health, illness, and life processes are subjective and qualitative research is the most feasible method of obtaining information and understanding of the human condition. In addition, sensitive measurement instruments that assess and document the interactive nature of each client's biological, psychological, emotional, sociological, and spiritual patterns are needed as well as ongoing evaluation of nursing interventions assessing their usefulness in promoting wellness and preventing illness.

The body of knowledge that frames holistic nursing includes knowledge of the science and understanding of the art of the profession. AHNA supports nursing research and scholarship that build scientific knowledge through empirical work and that extend humanistic understanding through qualitative investigations and creative expressions. AHNA endorses and supports nursing scholarship relevant to learning, documenting, and comprehending that which is the science and art of holistic nursing, with the goal of producing dependable and relevant information to practitioners and the public.

Revised and re-approved by ANHA, 2012.

White Paper: Research in AHNA

Rorry Zahourek, Ruth McCaffery, Sue Robertson, Evelyn Clingerman

Contributions: Marlaine Smith, Diane Wardell

This white paper will address AHNA's position on Holistic Nursing Research (HNR) and the organization's goals and strategies with respect to holistic nursing research. This will provide holistic nursing researchers with a platform on which to develop research. **This statement augments the description of holistic nursing research that is in the AHNA handbook. This statement is also in concert with the 2007 Standards of Holistic Nursing Practice.**

Nursing encompasses a body of knowledge focusing on human health and healing, through caring (Smith, 1994) or caring in the human health experience (Newman, Sime, & Corcoran-Perry, 1990). Within this framework, the person is considered to be whole and complete in the moment, and intimately connected to, and integral with, the environment. Person and environment are always in a mutual process of relationship. Every facet of this person-environment dynamic impacts the health and well-being of the person-family-community in all ways. Therefore, holistic nurses embrace culture, psychosocial influences, the physical environment, energetic principles, and spirituality as inseparable from physical manifestation of health and illness. Theory development related to the person-environment must be explored conceptually and empirically through research to enhance our knowledge of wholeness, health and healing, holistic caring, healing presence, and therapeutic connection.

Inquiry is the essence of all science. Holistic scientific inquiry and research emphasize the study of complexity of unitary patterning. Research explores phenomena central to the concern of holistic nurses. Holistic Nursing Research contributes to the growing evidence of the efficacy and safety of interventions so that they may be used judiciously.

Inherent in a holistic framework is the belief in, and experience of, working together with persons to integrate the use of modalities that may influence or promote the person's ability to manage and change health and illness patterns. Holistic care often includes the use of integrative and complementary, and/or alternative approaches, but those approaches always occur within the context of valuing persons and their community as a unitary whole and the use of therapeutic presence in the healing process. Solid evidence for the effectiveness of these approaches is often dependent on the interplay of relationships, the passage of time, and interaction of many variables some of which are not easily controlled for or measured using standard methods or a conventional scientific framework. As a result, research is often challenging and the questions posed may not always lend themselves to traditional designs such as the double-blind randomized controlled trials. In general, the strongest and most appropriate design and methods for research question posed should be employed. Results may need to be interpreted in functional and practical ways that apply to all areas of HN practice.

For example, understanding the effect of an intervention on the whole person often requires describing and evaluating feelings, sensations, and responses. Some holistic research aims to learn and understand the meaning of an experience as well as how the individual's personal essence and subtle energy fields are influenced. These are not easily measured in the quantitative realm. To capture the nature and effect of holistic interventions, various forms of qualitative research methods are often used. While qualitative evidence differs from the quantitative evidence produced by clinical trials, it is no less powerful in providing an understanding of the whole person. Holistic nursing uses a variety of research approaches including the standard double-blind randomized controlled clinical trial research method. However, it is more likely to combine approaches to provide evidence of the efficacy of holistic approaches to enhancing quality of life, health and well being. Therefore, additional methods to collect and analyze data are encouraged. These include various combinations of approaches, multiple site research projects, and aesthetic and creative methods.

Definition: Holistic nursing research includes:

- Extending, testing, and revising current theory and developing new theory

- Investigating the processes and efficacy of interventions

- Describing life experiences

- Exploring holistic nursing practice

- Comparison of groups, communities, or cultures.

An important caveat: To be "holistic" nursing research, the theoretical basis and interpretation of results must be within the context of holism. The AHNA recognizes two definitions of holism. Integrating one, or developing a unique definition of holism should be evident in the research question(s) study design, method, analysis, and interpretation of findings. The definition of holistic nursing as stated in the Leadership Council Handbook is as follows:

Holistic nursing embraces all nursing which has as its goal the enhancement of healing the whole person from birth to death. Holistic nursing recognizes that there are two views regarding holism: that holism involves identifying the interrelationships of the bio-psycho-social-spiritual dimensions of the person, recognizing that the whole is greater than the sum of its parts; and that holism involves understanding the individual as a unitary whole in mutual process with the environment. Holistic nursing responds to both views, believing that the goals of nursing can be achieved within either framework.

To facilitate the healing process and for nurses to become therapeutic partners with individuals, families, and communities, holistic nursing practice draws on nursing knowledge, theories, research, expertise, intuition, and creativity. Holistic nursing practice encourages peer review of professional practice in various clinical settings and integrates knowledge of current professional standards, laws, and regulations governing nursing practice" (LC Handbook, p., 6 2006).

The AHNA Research Committee's **overall purpose** is to promote holistic nursing research which includes: supporting select projects, developing projects, informing members about new and potentially useful research findings, providing support, education and mentoring to those desiring help developing or completing projects, and promoting community awareness of the value of HN research.

Holistic Nursing Research Goals

- Promote HN research in various clinical practice settings that advocate health and well-being.

- Partner with established research institutions to determine what are important research issues and problems, and to share human and material resources.

- Investigate key phenomena of concern related to HN.

- Expand the body of holistic nursing knowledge related to theory, practice, and education for both health care providers as well as the public.

- Clarify the nature and scope of HNR and develop expertise in, and expand the boundaries of, holistic nursing research.

- Encourage the use of an evidence-based nursing practice in which multiple forms of evidence are considered useful and significant.

- Encourage and educate nurses in the interpretation and use of research findings from various sources.

- Encourage and mentor holistic nurses in developing quality research studies.

- Provide HNR content in order to integrate concepts of holistic nursing research throughout their curriculum.

- Develop a call for research proposals to discover how holistic nursing research might be different from other specialty areas of research and nursing research.

Strategies

- Foster programs to educate nurses about holistic nursing research including web-based tutorials.

- Using the AHNA network, develop a consultation and a mentor program for nurses who want to do holistic nursing research.

- Begin to collect holistic nursing research and contribute that to the web library. Establish a repository of holistic nursing research.

- Develop a multisite research project that has sufficient funds to support staff and researchers and is grounded in the theme *Healing through Holistic Nursing*.

- Continue to fund small research projects done by AHNA members.

- Promote means to utilize and integrate holistic nursing research into education and practice.

- Provide schools of nursing with examples of holistic nursing research.

- Develop a call for holistic nursing research proposals that differentiate holistic nursing from other specialty groups.

- Develop more sources of outside funding; partner with agencies and/or schools of nursing who already have funding and an interest and commitment re holistic nursing practice.

- Include research-related workshops at yearly conferences.

With an increased public interest in and understanding of mind-body-spirit connections, the potential usefulness of complementary-integrative and emerging modalities, and the interconnectedness of a global community, there is need for evidence-based nursing practice related to holistic nursing care. Various approaches to health, healing, and the management of illness have expanded and are being increasingly sought by the American public. To meet this need, expanded and more flexible methods and creative approaches to research are required.

Submitted March, 2009. Approved by the Leadership Council April, 2009.
Rorry Zahourek, PhD, PMHCNS-BC, AHN-BC
Coordinator for Research
AHNA

Index

Note: An entry with [2007] indicates it is from *Holistic Nursing: Scope and Standards of Practice* (2007), reproduced in Appendix A. That information is not current but is included for historical value only.

A

Accountability in holistic nursing, x

Acupressure, 13–14

Acupuncture, 26

Acute care hospitals, 21

Advanced Holistic Nurse, Board Certified (AHN-BC), 27

Advanced Practice Holistic Nurse Certification examination (APHN-BC, APRN), 27

Advanced practice registered nurses in holistic nursing practice (APRNs), 24–25
  assessment competencies, 51
  certification, 27
  collaboration competencies, 80
  communication competencies, 75
  consultation competencies, 62,
  continuing education, 24–24
  coordination of care competencies, 59
  diagnosis competencies, 52
  education competencies, 69
  ethics competencies, 67
  evaluation competencies, 65

  evidence-based practice and research competencies, 71
  environmental health competencies, 84–85
  health teaching and health promotion competencies, 61
  implementation competencies, 58
  leadership competencies, 77–78
  outcomes identification competencies, 54
  planning competencies, 56
  prescriptive authority competencies, 63
  professional practice evaluation competencies, 81
  quality of practice competencies, 73
  resource utilization competencies, 83

Aging, defined, 29

AHNA. *See* American Holistic Nurses Association (AHNA)

AHNCC. *See* American Holistic Nurses Certification Corporation (AHNCC)

Alexander Technique, 13

Allopathic/conventional therapies, defined, 87